MITRAL VALVE PROLAPSE

Mitral Valve Prolapse

Robert M. Jeresaty, M.D.

Director
Section of Cardiology
Saint Francis Hospital and Medical Center
and
Associate Professor of Medicine
University of Connecticut School of Medicine
Hartford, Connecticut

Raven Press ▪ New York

Raven Press, 1140 Avenue of the Americas, New York, New York 10036

Made in the United States of America

Library of Congress Cataloging in Publication Data

Jeresaty, Robert M.
  Mitral valve prolapse.

  Includes bibliographical references and index.
  1. Mitral valve--Displacement. I. Title. [DNLM:
1. Mitral valve insufficiency. 2. Prolapse. WG262
J55m]
RC685.V2J47   616.1'25   78-66350
ISBN 0-89004-230-6

To my wife Cathie and my children
Denise, Michael, Joseph, Nadine, and Joanne,
and to my parents, Dr. and Mrs. Michel Jeresaty

Preface

The mitral valve prolapse-click syndrome, no longer considered a benign curiosity, continues to generate great interest. It is the most common cardiac valve disorder. The numerous papers and presentations devoted to it during the past 10 years would probably qualify it as the cardiac disease of the decade. In spite of the outpouring of publications on the syndrome, much of the information remains incomplete, often contradictory, and frequently controversial. It is now generally accepted that the click and the associated late systolic murmur are mitral in origin. Several features of this syndrome are responsible, in particular, for the widespread attention it is receiving: its prevalence, its controversial etiology, and the clinical features that it shares with coronary artery disease such as chest pain, ST-T changes, and arrhythmias. An auscultatory "silent" variety has recently been identified, and an advanced form, "the floppy mitral valve," has been established as a major cause of mitral insufficiency. Echocardiography, a widely used noninvasive technique that has joined auscultation and angiocardiography as a third major diagnostic marker in this syndrome, has catalyzed the current information explosion.

My own interest in this syndrome dates back to the mid 1960s. Over the years, I have collected a series of 350 cases. During the past 2 years, I have included only unusual cases in my series. In the early 1970s, I sought to draw the attention of cardiologists to the prevalence of this syndrome and to dissociate it from coronary artery disease. I provided a detailed description of its angiographic signs and described an auscultatory "silent" form of this syndrome. Although the published reports and my own studies suggest that myxomatous transformation of the mitral valve is probably the underlying pathological disorder, the etiology and the nature of the myxomatous changes remain a puzzle.

The prevalence of this syndrome and its obscure etiology have encouraged the publication of multiple reports on its association with other entities ranging from coronary artery disease and rheumatic heart disease to hypertrophic subaortic stenosis and acromegaly. It is my contention that this association is coincidental and casual rather than causal. Until more evidence is presented, the "purists" should resist the assaults of the "associationists" who tend to confuse the etiological picture of this syndrome. "Associationists" have been encouraged by the finding of angiographic prolapse in various entities. The nonejection click, however, remains the characteristic auscultatory hallmark of idiopathic mitral valve prolapse and should allow us to differentiate it from secondary angiographic prolapse, a less specific finding. Despite its short-comings, echocardiography is of great value in the identification of idiopathic mitral valve prolapse.

The purpose of this book is to review the etiology, pathology, and symptomatology of this syndrome, as well as its auscultatory, phonocardiographic, electrocardiographic, echocardiographic, and angiographic features. Its infrequent complications (e.g., ruptured chordae tendineae, infective endocarditis, and sudden death) are discussed. On the basis of published works and my own observations, I propose theories to explain the various aspects of this syndrome. It is hoped that this book will help clarify the confusing picture that emerges from the literature and that causes some physicians either to overdiagnose this syndrome or to deny its existence altogether. I seek to describe a framework that will allow a more meaningful research into the etiology, significance, and features of this fascinating syndrome.

Robert M. Jeresaty, M.D.

Acknowledgments

This monograph is an expression of the interest in mitral valve prolapse of the Section of Cardiology at Saint Francis Hospital and Medical Center, Hartford, Connecticut. It embodies the cooperative effort of many cardiologists, notably Dr. Joseph P. Liss, Dr. Arthur B. Landry, Jr., Dr. Subrata K. Basu, Dr. H. Robert Silverstein, Dr. Joseph B. Sappington, Dr. David J. O'Reilly, and Dr. Russell A. Ciafone. I wish to acknowledge the contributions of these cardiologists and of our cardiac fellows to the study of the 350 patients with MVP followed by our group. I am also most grateful for the support and encouragement of Sister Francis Marie, Executive Director of our institution, Dr. Stephen B. Sulavik, former Director of Medicine, and Dr. J. David Schnatz, our present Director of Medicine.

Dr. Arnold M. Katz, Professor and Chief of the Division of Cardiology, University of Connecticut School of Medicine, has played the role of a catalyst in my decision to write this monograph. Having just completed his excellent monograph, *Physiology of the Heart,* he urged me to write a book on mitral valve prolapse and was instrumental in putting me in touch with Raven Press, the publishers of both of our monographs. His encouragement and his contagious enthusiasm are greatly appreciated.

I am dedicating this book to my wife and to my children who have tolerated endless evening and weekend hours of painstaking preparation and who have looked upon my endeavor as a "family enterprise." I was constantly sustained and exhorted by their repeated query, "What page are you on?" If the answer denoted a slow pace, it never failed to elicit the enthusiastic response of "fantastic" from our seven-year-old Joanne. My wife, Cathie, has contributed numerous and exhausting hours to the typing and retyping of parts of the manuscript, and to the organization of the illustrations and the references. This book is also dedicated to my loving mother and to my father, who remains for me a living example of perfectionism, organization, and dedication to the medical profession.

I am greatly indebted to Mrs. Dorothea Murray for her valuable secretarial assistance. The expert help of Mrs. Joy Scavotto, our echocardiographic technician, is acknowledged, as well as the enthusiastic contribution of Mrs. Kathleen Walsh to the recording of the phonocardiograms. I wish also to thank Ms. Ruth Carroll, our Director of Libraries, and her dedicated staff for their help in the review of the medical literature and in obtaining the needed references. Mr. Frank Sullo and his assistant, Mr. Joseph Milhomens, have provided expert photographic assistance and have graciously responded to unreasonable demands.

Finally, I wish to thank Raven Press and especially Dr. Diana M. Schneider, Ms. Virginia B. Martin, and Ms. Terry Kornak for their invaluable cooperation and their help in editing and polishing this text.

R. M. J.

Contents

Chapter 1

History and Terminology

HISTORICAL BACKGROUND

The midsystolic click, first described in 1887 as a "bruit" de galop mésosystolique" (88) was thought by Gallavardin to be extracardiac and due to pleuropericardial adhesions (136). However, in 1931 White suggested that the midsystolic sounds were mitral in origin and arose from abnormal chordae tendineae (379). In 1935, Thompson and Levine (360) reported on a clinical investigation of 35 patients with "systolic gallop rhythm." They described many features that were subsequently rediscovered: prevalence, occurrence in "nervous people," variable intensity, and evanescence of the click, chest discomfort and palpitations. They stressed the generally benign nature of the systolic gallop rhythm when compared to diastolic gallop and stated that "It has no unfavorable influence on prognosis."

In 1880, Osler described the systolic whoop but did not ascribe it to the mitral valve (265). Although Griffith in 1892 (147) had suggested that an apical mid-to-late systolic murmur might be due to mitral regurgitation, this murmur was regarded as innocent (161,214) until the early 1960s. In 1962, Humphries and McKusick (161), who postulated a pericardial origin of the click, described the association of the midsystolic click, late systolic murmur and T wave changes and coined the term "auscultatory-electrocardiographic syndrome."

Gallavardin's hypothesis was unchallenged until Reid (298), in 1961, proposed a mitral valvular origin for the click and the murmur and ascribed the click to sudden tensing of the chordae, "chordal snap." Barlow et al. (18,20) deserve credit for having shown that the association of click, late systolic murmur, a distinctive electrocardiographic pattern, and angiographic mitral valve prolapse constitutes a specific syndrome.

Reid and Barlow's hypothesis was subsequently confirmed on the basis of the following evidence: (a) The late systolic murmur behaved like the murmur of mitral regurgitation, decreasing in intensity with amyl nitrite inhalation and increasing with phenylephrine infusion (18). (b) Mitral regurgitation was visualized angiographically in patients with late systolic murmur (20). (c) Both click and late systolic murmur were recorded in the left atrium with intracardiac phonocardiography using a phono-catheter passed through the lumen of a transeptal catheter (218,311). (d) Mitral valve prolapse was demonstrated angiographically in patients with clicks

1

and/or late systolic murmurs (17,171,197). (e) The click was recorded at the time of maximal billowing of the posterior leaflet (85). (f) Prolapse of the mitral leaflet was noted on echocardiography in patients with clicks and late systolic murmurs (109,191).

Hancock and Cohn's description of the clinical features of this syndrome was a classic in clinical research (154). Several large series were subsequently reported (175,276,322,339) and various surveys were carried out attesting to the prevalence of this syndrome. Its angiographic (175,197) and echocardiographic features (99,282) have been well described in various reports.

TERMINOLOGY

Various terms and names have been proposed to designate this syndrome (Table 1.1). Barlow (276) coined the terms *billowing posterior mitral leaflet syndrome* and *nonejection clicks*. I am guilty of having used two terms adding to the terminology confusion in the literature: *the syndrome associated with midsystolic click and/or late systolic murmur* (169) and *ballooning of the mitral valve leaflets* (171) before settling on *mitral valve prolapse–click syndrome* (175). Criley et al. (85) were probably the first to use *prolapse of the mitral valve* (85) to describe this syndrome. In the American literature, mitral valve prolapse (MVP) is now generally accepted as the standard designation of this syndrome, justifying, in my opinion, the plea for unanimity made by Abrams (3). The term *non-ejection click* seems most appropriate to designate the systolic click in this syndrome. The timing of the click (early, mid or late systolic) is variable and should not be used to identify the auscultatory component of this syndrome. The non-ejection click is the characteristic hallmark of this syndrome and, despite its occurrence in pneumothorax, in a rare case of atrial myxoma and in congenital aneurysm of the interventricular septum, it constitutes a specific sign of idiopathic MVP. An isolated late systolic murmur, however, is a nonspecific auscultatory finding and requires echocardiographic or angiographic confirmation before ascribing it to mitral valve prolapse. Angiographic mitral

TABLE 1.1 *The most commonly used terms to designate the mitral valve prolapse syndrome*

Click syndrome	Prolapsing mitral leaflet syndrome
Click murmur syndrome	Mitral valve prolapse
Systolic click-late systolic mumur syndrome	Idiopathic mitral valve prolapse
	Mitral valve prolapse syndrome
Billowing posterior leaflet syndrome	Mitral valve prolapse-click syndrome
	Auscultatory-electrocardiographic syndrome
Ballooning of the mitral valve leaflets	"Floppy" valve syndrome
	"Click chick" syndrome
Overshooting mitral leaflets	
Barlow's syndrome	

prolapse is less specific than the click for the diagnosis of MVP syndrome. The same angiographic picture has been described in idiopathic MVP, in coronary artery disease, and in hypertrophic subaortic stenosis. Therefore, the finding of mitral leaflet prolapse on left ventriculography in patients with known coronary artery disease does not warrant the additional diagnosis of MVP unless a click is heard or the echocardiogram is confirmatory.

The posterior mitral valve leaflet is not exclusively involved in MVP and this syndrome should not, therefore, be designated as prolapse, ballooning, or billowing of the posterior leaflet.

In view of the acceptance of the term *mitral valve prolapse* and its meaning, the specificity of the click and the nonspecificity of the late systolic murmur and the angiographic findings, the likelihood that myxomatous degeneration of the mitral cusps is the underlying pathological lesion in this entity, I would propose that one of the following terms be used to designate this syndrome: (a) Mitral valve prolapse-click syndrome or (b) Idiopathic or primary (84) mitral valve prolapse. If a click is heard, the former designation is appropriate. However, in the absence of a click ("silent" form, late systolic or pansystolic murmur with angiographic and/or echocardiographic confirmation) the latter designation should be used (See Chap. 4 for further comment on this concept).

The term *floppy mitral valve* should be reserved for the advanced form of this syndrome that is associated with pansystolic murmur and severe mitral insufficiency.

Chapter 2

Prevalence, Sex and Age Distribution

Idiopathic MVP is probably the most common valve disease in adults. Several large series (175,231,276,322) attest to its prevalence. My own series currently consists of 350 patients. A nonejection click confirmed by phonocardiography or, in the absence of a click, MVP proven by left ventriculography and in most patients by echocardiography, were a prerequisite for patients to be included in my series. Echocardiography was not used, therefore, as the sole diagnostic marker in my series. In a survey of 1,169 wives of Air Force personnel examined during a "Womens Health Week," Procacci et al. (286) reported a prevalence of 6.3% (Table 2.1). Unfortunately, they have not confirmed their findings by phonocardiography, but their patients were examined on multiple occasions by at least three of the authors and echocardiography corroborated the auscultatory diagnosis in 80% of these subjects; only 8% of their MVP patients had the nonspecific late systolic murmur. Brown et al. (45) after echocardiographically surveying 520 women and 180 men reported the same figure of 6% in women, and a much lower figure of 0.5% in men; the echocardiographic findings were usually supported by the presence of a systolic click (23 out of 29 females with positive echocardiograms). A slightly lower figure of 4.4% was reported by Block et al. (36) using stringent echocardiographic criteria (e.g., midsystolic displacement or pansystolic sagging of 5 mm or more) in a study of 136 normal volunteers. A much higher incidence (17%) was reported by Markiewicz et al. (233), but the women surveyed by these authors answered newspaper advertisements of the type that may attract individuals suffering from the cardiopulmonary symptoms or the psychoneurotic disorders frequently encountered in this syndrome. Lower prevalence had been reported by Rizzon et al. (302) in an auscultatory–phonocardiographic survey of 1,003 female students aged 14 to 24 (0.4%) and by McLaren et al. (249) in a much larger auscultatory survey of 12,050 children in Soweto, South Africa (1.4%) but without phonocardiographic confirmation. In a communication to the author, Dr. Barlow (16) stated, "This prevalence of 1.4% is far too low! We have done a more careful survey (not yet published) and I was a little disappointed and surprised to hear clicks in ± 17%." Dr Barlow did not provide a breakdown of the auscultatory findings in his cases. The high prevalence of rheumatic fever in the South African black population would explain, in my opinion, the high prevalence of the nonspecific late systolic murmur in these children.

TABLE 2.1. *Prevalence of idiopathic mvp*

Source of data	Population size	% of prolapse
Rizzon (302)	1009[a]	0.33
Brown (45)	520[a]	1.4
Markiewicz (233)	100[a]	17.0
Procacci (286)	1169[a]	6.3
McLaren (249)	12050[b]	1.4
Barlow (16)	unknown	17.0
Block (36)	136	4.4
Longo (227)	900[c]	1.5

[a] female population
[b] children
[c] aircrewmen

There is a comparatively high prevalence (1%) of myxomatous degeneration of one or both cusps in general hospital necropsy material in adult patients (279).

The true prevalence of idiopathic MVP in the general population has not been established yet, and the results of various surveys are variable. The 6% figure reported by Procacci et al. and Brown et al. is probably the most accurate for a young female population. In view of the known female preponderance, a 4% prevalence in the general population can be extrapolated.

Methodology for further surveys should probably abide by the following rules:

1. The population surveyed should not be recruited through advertisements in newspapers.
2. The auscultatory findings should be confirmed by phonocardiography.
3. Late systolic murmur should not be considered as a sign of prolapse in the absence of echocardiographic confirmation.
4. Echocardiography, in view of the variability of its criteria, should not be used as the sole method of detection of prolapse except when midsystolic buckling is used as the diagnostic marker.

The high prevalence of nonejection clicks in the general population and the lack of symptoms in most subjects who have a click have caused some workers to question the existence of the MVP syndrome (153). This reasoning, if pursued to the extreme, should make us doubt the existence of hypertension (which has a prevalence of 10% in the general population), of coronary artery disease etc. because they are prevalent and most patients affected by these diseases are free of symptoms, particularly in the early stages. While acknowledging the high prevalence of idiopathic MVP and the benign asymptomatic course of most patients afflicted, I believe that it is logical to look upon it as a syndrome with a wide spectrum ranging from the asymptomatic to the severely disabling forms. The mechanism of the development of symptoms in a relatively small number of these patients remains unexplained.

A female preponderance has been reported in this syndrome (154,175, 231,249,276) (Table 2.2), women constituting approximately two-thirds of

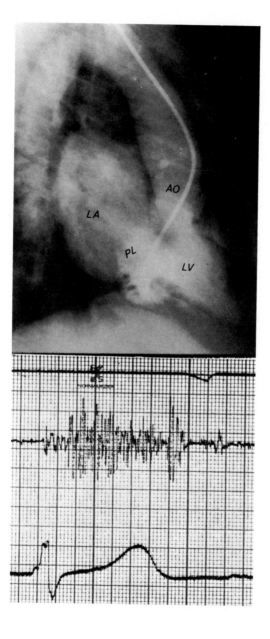

FIG. 2.1. Case 35. Angiogram and phonocardiogram of a 2½-year-old boy. Left ventricular angiogram in the lateral position shows prolapse of posteromedial and middle scallop of the posterior leaflet (PL), moderately severe to severe mitral insufficiency, and dilatation of the ascending aorta (AO). LA, left atrium; LV, Left ventricle. Phonocardiogram: pansystolic murmur and third heart sound. EKG: left anterior hemiblock. No shunts were noted on catheterization. (From ref. 171 By permission)

TABLE 2.2. *Sex distribution of mvp*

Source of data	Patients surveyed	% of women
Pocock (276)	130	72
Jeresaty (175)	100	64
Malcolm (231)	85	58
Hancock (154)	45	58
McLaren (249)	168	65

patients with idiopathic MVP. A preponderance of males over females has been described in patients with pansystolic murmurs and in those with infective endocarditis (80).

The mean age was about 40 (154,231,276) with a range of 2 to 84 years. This syndrome has been reported in children (Figs. 2.1 and 12.8). However, except in surveys conducted in Soweto, Johannesburg (16,249) a relative paucity of cases in this age group is noted, particularly in the familial form (18,115,144,154,162,175,197,315,324,325,334,345). This observation suggests that although this syndrome may be genetically determined, its manifestations do not usually become evident before adulthood. A recent report on surgical treatment of "floppy" mitral valve in five children ranging in age from 9 to 14 years, commented on the exceptionally rapid deterioration in congestive heart failure in this age group after onset of symptoms.

Most of the reported cases have been white patients; however, this syndrome also occurs in Blacks: 13% of my first 100 cases were Black (175) and McClaren et al. (249) reported a 1.4% prevalence of this syndrome in the Black population of Soweto.

FAMILIAL PREVALENCE AND GENETIC TRANSMISSON OF MVP

The familial occurrence of this syndrome was described in various series (19,139,162,276,302,332,334,347,376). Shell et al. (53) reported on four families with this syndrome in addition to six gathered from the literature. A family in whom 11 members had clinical features of MVP was described by Hunt et al. (162). Barlow and Pocock (276) encountered a total of 85 patients involving 26 families (19). Utilizing echocardiography, Weiss et al. (376) studied 74 subjects composed of 17 propositi with MVP and 57 first degree relatives. MVP was detected in 47% (27 of 57) of the first degree relatives. Familial transmission occurred from propositi to both sexes. Fifty-three percent of females and 36% of male progeni of propositi were affected. A greater percentage of transmission from mothers of propositi (7 of 9) was also noted. In a similar study of 59 first degree relatives of 18 index patients, Scheele et al (324) reported a lower familial prevalence of 30.5%

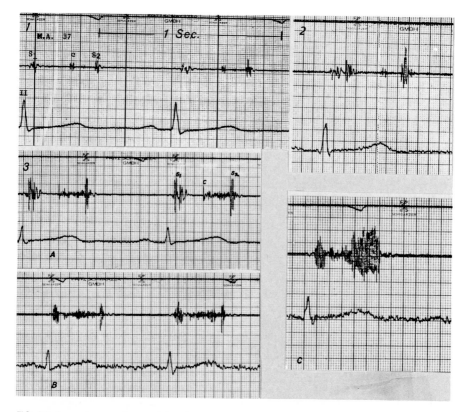

FIG. 2.2. Apex phonocardiogram (phono) in two identical twins and their mother. 1. Case 83. 2 MSC (c) are recorded. 2. Case 76. Daughter aged 17: an early click and two MSC are evident. Early diastolic murmur of aortic insufficiency. 3. Case 77. Daughter aged 17: A. Supine: MSC and LSM. B. Standing position: Pansystolic murmur and questionable early click. C. Left decubitus position: "Honk" and early click. (From ref. 175 By permission)

(18 out of 59). The echocardiographic evidence of MVP was 50% (9 out of 18) in the parents of the index subjects, 29% (7 of 24) in their siblings, and only 11.8% (2 of 17) in their children. When the first degree relatives were evaluated by age group, 46% (13 of 28) aged more than 20 years and only 16% (5 of 31) aged less than 20 years had MVP.

An autosomal form of inheritance with incomplete penetrance and reduced expressivity in the male and the young was demonstrated (162,324,334, 376). No chromosome abnormalities were reported (347).

I have not carried out extensive family studies. In my series, familial occurrence was noted in nine instances including the first report of this syndrome in identical twins in the absence of Marfan's syndrome (175) (Fig. 2.2). I have recently observed two other sets of identical twins in whom the diagnosis of idiopathic MVP was made. The occurrence of MVP in twins has been reported in two other instances (139,302) with echocardiographic diagnosis of MVP in one of the two sets of twins (139).

Chapter 3

Pathological Findings

Fernex and Fernex (126) were the first to describe prolapsed myxomatous mitral valve leaflets and to ascribe significant mitral regurgitation to the myxomatous changes. Read et al. (297) coined the expression *floppy valve syndrome* in reporting their findings in six patients with myxomatous valvular transformation. Other workers have described the anatomical features of this syndrome (4,32,46,54,57,63,73,75,77,91,108,126,143,150,157,158,175,192, 193,199,212,223,229,232,243,244,253,278,291,297,304,306,317,328,335, 336,364,370,380,393). Because of the generally benign course of idiopathic MVP, the underlying pathology in this syndrome has been mainly documented in the advanced cases who had a pansystolic murmur, underwent surgery for severe mitral regurgitation, or succumbed as a result of their valve disease. Of great interest, from an etiological viewpoint, has been the demonstration of the same pathological changes in 26 patients with isolated nonejection clicks or with clicks followed by a late systolic murmur (18,19, 73,75,80,91,115,139,150,157,179,192,229,239,243,253,277,282,304,319, 332,370,376). To my knowledge, no cases of "silent" MVP have come to surgery or necropsy.

Documented anatomical features include the following:

1. Voluminous redundant, scalloped and thickened leaflets.
2. Mitral annular dilatation.
3. Myxomatous transformation of the valve substance.
4. Absence of inflammatory changes.
5. Absence of small coronary arteriopathy.

LEAFLETS AND CHORDAE TENDINEAE

The leaflets are redundant and present a hooded appearance, convex toward the left atrium (Figs. 3.1–3.4). The domed leaflets and scallops and their chordae resemble a parachute (279). The loss of the collagenous supporting structure of the valve allows stretching of the cusps by the ventricular pressure and results in hooded, prolapsed leaflets. However, the distinction between minimal prolapse as a "variant of the normal" and abnormal prolapse is not readily made on inspection of the mitral valve (336). Shrivastava et al. (336) pointed out that interchordal hooding occurs normally because chordal insertions into the leaflets are focal. To quote the same authors, "Considering that the normal leaflet is delicate, it is to be ex-

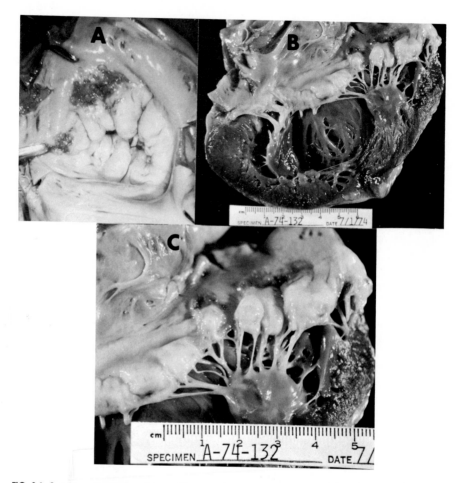

FIG. 3.1. Specimens from a female, age 39, who died suddenly in 1974. Multiple clicks and a late systolic murmur were heard and recorded in 1965. A. Mitral valve seen from the left atrium. Marked redundancy, hooding and ballooning of both anterior and posterior leaflets. Ulceration at junction of posterior leaflet and left atrium. No vegetations were noted. B. Hooding of anterior leaflet and of triscalloped posterior leaflet. Chordae intact, thickened and shortened. C. Close-up view of the redundant mitral leaflet. (From ref. 181 By permission)

pected that as left ventricular systolic pressure is applied to the leaflet, there will be some prolapse toward the left atrium of those leaflet elements that lie between chordal insertion."

A wide spectrum of leaflet abnormalities has been described (175,306) ranging from grade 1 on a scale of 4 (histological changes with grossly normal leaflets) to grade 2 (prolapse without mitral regurgitation) and grade 3 (prolapse with mild mitral regurgitation) to grade 4 (prolapse with moderate to severe mitral regurgitation) (Fig. 3.5).

The chordae tendineae are typically elongated and thin (108,332) but may be thickened (380). The abnormally increased length of the chordae may be the result of mucinous alteration of these structures but is probably a

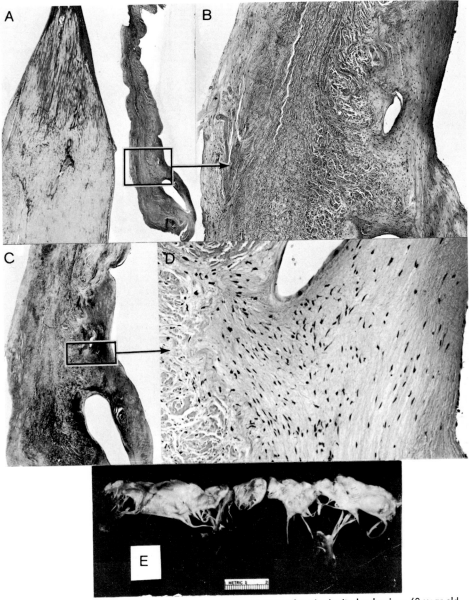

FIG. 3.2. *Case 43.* Histologic sections and gross appearance of excised mitral valve in a 69-year-old man. A. Included here is the apical portion of one papillary muscle as well as a portion of the anterior mitral leaflet. Some scarring is present in the apex of the papillary muscle. The leaflet is thickened. B. A close-up of the area in brackets is shown. The thickening is due primarily to the presence of a myxoid stroma containing large amounts of acid mucopolysaccharide (AMP) material. C. A close-up of one area of the leaflet shown in B. This is an AMP stain. The darker area represents large collections of AMP. D. Close-up of area shown in C. This area contains strap cells surrounded by strongly AMP positive material. Rinehart stains, ×4.5 (A); ×15 (C); hematocylin and eosin stains, ×30 (B); ×120 (D). E. Excised mitral valve showing redundancy and ballooning of the anterior leaflet and three scallops of the posterior leaflet. See left cineventriculogram in Fig. 12.16. (Courtesy of Dr. William C. Roberts and from ref. 175 By permission)

consequence of abnormal tension upon them by the prolapsing leaflets (150). The chordae may become thickened as a reaction to friction against the endocardium, fusion, and coalescence (150). The adhesion of chordae to the

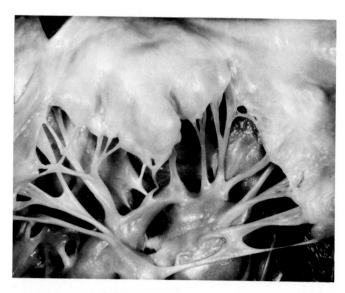

FIG. 3.3. Myxomatous mitral valve from a 29-year-old man who died suddenly. Note characteristic inter-chordal hooding and variation in the thickness of the chordae. (Courtesy of Drs. Jesse E. Edwards and Richard B. Guthrie. From ref. 150 by permission)

mural endocardium may result in effective shortening of initially long chordae (150).

Earlier studies stressed the exclusive involvement of the posterior mitral leaflet in this syndrome (17). Predominant involvement of the posterior leaflet has been observed by the Toronto group and others (150,380). In

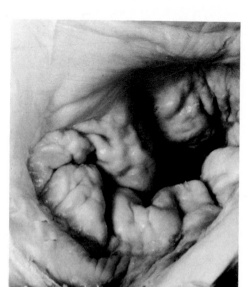

FIG. 3.4. Prolapsed and redundant mitral valve viewed from above. (Courtesy of Dr. Jesse E. Edwards).

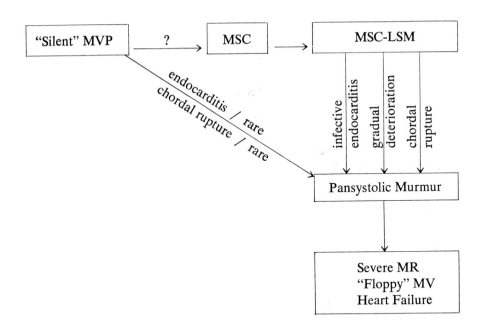

FIG. 3.5. The spectrum and possible natural history of MVP. The auscultatory mode of presentation is de-picted in this figure. The various auscultatory forms share the same echocardiographic and angiographic features of MVP. They also share the same pathological lesions with variable severity. However, patholog-ical studies in "silent" MVP have not been reported yet. Progression from one subset to the other has been documented in only a few cases (See Chap. 14). MSC, midsystolic click; LSM, late systolic murmur; MR, mitral regurgitation. Modified from ref. 307.

1973, I reviewed the pathological and surgical literature and found that identification of the deformed leaflet was provided in 46 cases with prolapse of the posterior leaflet in 15, of the anterior in 4, and of both leaflets in 27 (175) (Figs. 3.1 and 3.3). Therefore, both leaflets are usually involved and, to quote Popp et al. (282), "The abnormal process does not stop at the commissures of the valve." In patients with either prolapse of anterior leaflets or prolapse of both leaflets a higher incidence of severe mitral regurgitation were described (175). It is possible that mildly symptomatic patients with nonejection clicks and absent or insignificant mitral regurgitation have iso-lated or predominant prolapse of the posterior leaflet.

MORPHOLOGY OF THE POSTERIOR MITRAL LEAFLET

Ranganathan et al. (291) showed that the posterior leaflet of the mitral valve is divided into scallops by clefts, being triscalloped in 46 of 50 hearts studied (Figs. 3.2 and 3.3). In 42 hearts a large middle scallop was present with two small commissural scallops, the posteromedial and the anterolateral on either side. Either an anterolateral or a posteromedial scallop was the largest in the other four hearts. The appreciation of this triscalloped morphology has been most helpful in the angiographic and echocardiographic diagnosis of mitral valve prolapse (175).

MITRAL ANNULAR DILATATION

Mitral annular dilatation has been described in this syndrome (46,212). Bulkley and Roberts (46) showed that mitral annular dilatation that is excessive for a given degree of ventricular enlargement occurs only in subjects with MVP or Marfan's syndrome. The circumference of the mitral annulus in patients with normal hearts averaged 9 cm and only 11 cm in patients with idiopathic cardiomyopathy. In contrast, in patients with "floppy" valves with or without Marfan's syndrome, the annulus was greatly dilated (average 15.5 cm). These authors concluded that "abnormality of the fibrous skeleton of the heart is necessary for the mitral annulus to dilate enough to cause mitral regurgitation." Another interesting finding in this report is that of dilatation of the mitral annulus exceeding the size of the midportion of the left ventricle only in patients with "floppy" mitral valves with or without Marfan's syndrome. Dilatation of the annulus may explain some of the angiographic features of idiopathic MVP (See Chap. 12).

RUPTURE OF THE CHORDAE TENDINEAE

Rupture of the chordae tendineae is frequently associated with myxomatous mitral leaflets (150). (See Chap. 14). Studies of spontaneous chordal rupture has shown "that there is prolapse not only of the segment that has lost its chordal support but of other elements of the valve" (336). Moreover, fibrous endocardial lesions similar to those seen in idiopathic MVP have been noted (336).

INVOLVEMENT OF OTHER VALVES

Tricuspid valve prolapse has been documented by intracardiac phonocardiography, echocardiography, and angiography (4,63,143,158,232,322). In a review of the necropsy findings of 35 cases of ballooning deformity of the mitral valve, Pomerance (278) noted similar involvement in 9 tricuspid valves; these changes were described as mucoid degeneration. The same author, in a subsequent article (279), reported that the tricuspid valve is affected microscopically in approximately one-fourth of cases but the distortion is minor because of the lower pressures, and is of no clinical significance. In eight other cases, "floppy" tricuspid valves were noted at surgery (63,115) and on postmortem studies (54,57,193) in patients with "floppy" mitral valve. In one of these cases (57) the pulmonary valve was involved by the myxomatous process.

Myxomatous transformation of the aortic valve was described (193,244, 297) as an isolated lesion or in association with "floppy" mitral valve. In Read et al.'s (297) cases, the aortic insufficiency "appeared to be the result of prolapse of the leaflets which were "floppy" and lacked their normal form rigidity." In the clinical setting, association of aortic insufficiency with MVP is very uncommon (only 2 cases in our series), and is only noted in association with severe MVP, the "floppy" mitral valve syndrome.

ENDOCARDIAL AND MYOCARDIAL LESIONS

Fibrous lesions of the left ventricular endocardium with adhesions of the chordae and collagenous prolongation into the subjacent myocardium have been noted (278,317). Friction by the chordae that are unusually tensed by the hooded leaflet and abnormally close to the endocardium is considered the mechanism of these lesions (317). It is probable that abnormal tension on the papillary muscle and subsequent ischemia may be responsible for the fibrosis and scarring of this structure described in a few reports (Fig. 3.2) (364).

Using transvenous right ventricular endomyocardial septal biopsy on 12 patients with symptomatic click-murmur-mitral valve prolapse syndrome, Koch et al. (199) reported, in an abstract, "mild to moderate interstitial fibrosis in nine patients and mild to moderate endocardial fibrosis in four."

MYXOMATOUS TRANSFORMATION OF THE MITRAL VALVE

Myxomatous degeneration has been described as "disruption and loss of normal valvular architecture accompanied by an increase in ground substance with no appreciable inflammatory reaction" (242). There is an increased accumulation of acid mucopolysaccarides (AMP) composed of hyaluronic and/or chondroitin sulphate (223) (Fig. 3.2). It is not known if accumulation of AMP is due to a biochemical disorder of synthesis or of degradation. Staining methods for demonstration of myxomatous material include Alcian blue (pH 2.5), PAS with and without diastase digestion, AMP (colloidal iron) as modified by Rinehart with and without testicular hyaluronidase digestion (175,239,306). Alcian blue, PAS, and AMP strains are strongly positive.

The mitral valve, as do all valves, consists of two major components: the fibrosa and the spongiosa, which are surrounded by two thin layers: the auricularis on the atrial side and the ventricularis on the ventricular side (Fig. 3.6). The fibrosa, which is comprised of a sheet of dense collagen, forms the basic support of the leaflet and is continuous with the fibrous tissue of the annulus in the case of the posterior leaflet or the aortic–mitral intervalvular fibrosa in the case of the anterior leaflet. The spongiosa that is formed by myxomatous tissue lies between the auricularis and fibrosa layer

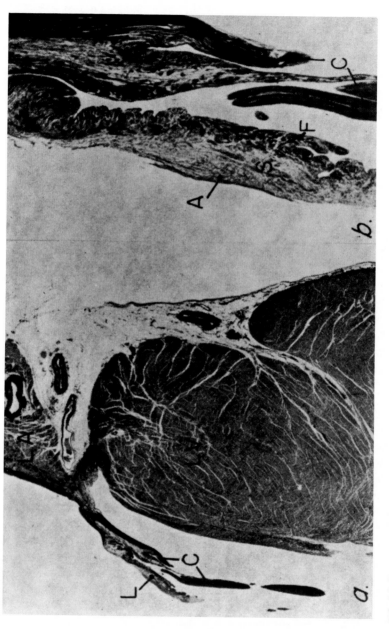

FIG. 3.6. Photomicrographs of normal mitral valve. A. Low power view of left atrium (LA) and left ventricle (LV) as well as the posterior mitral leaflet (L). Chordae (C) extend to the leaflet. Characteristically, the leaflet is thin. Elastic tissue stain; ×3.8 B. Segment of leaflet shown in (A). The leaflet is composed of the following layers: auricularis (A), spongiosa (S) and fibrosa (F). Chordae are indicated by letter C. Elastic tissue stain; ×20. (Courtesy of Drs. R. B. Guthrie and J. E. Edwards and by permission of *Minn Med*).

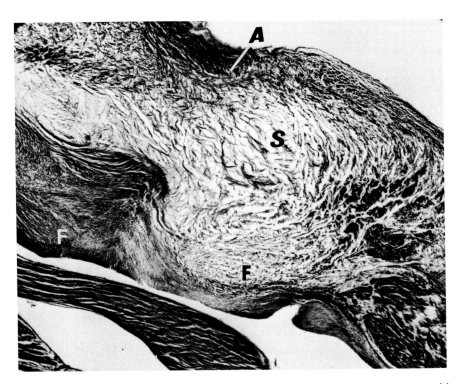

FIG. 3.7. Myxomatous mitral valve. The spongiosa (S) is voluminous and encroaches upon the fibrosa (F) and the auricularis (A). Elastic tissue stain; ×40. (Courtesy of Drs. R. B. Guthrie and J. E. Edwards and by permission of *Minn Med*).

(150). In most valvular heart disease, the spongiosa component is either partially or completely replaced by the proliferating fibrosa whereas in MVP the spongiosa, that portion of the valve that contains AMP material is the component that proliferates (150,304,306) (Fig. 3.7). This would explain the increased amount of AMP in "floppy" leaflets. The thickened spongiosa encroaches upon the fibrosa, interrupting it focally and causing a basic weakness of this supporting structure: "As the weakened leaflet is stretched by the pressure exerted upon it during left ventricular systole, it becomes deformed" (150). Roberts (304,306) objected to the use of the term *myxomatous degeneration* and to the description of the spongiosa as disorganized because there is no evidence that the AMP is degenerated and "little information regarding normal organization of the spongiosa is available for comparison." In a histologic study of 344 consecutive surgically excised valves (193), myxomatous transformation was noted in 262 users. However, in most cases, the myxomatous changes were minimal, being severe and disruptive in only 34 instances (10%). Lesser degrees of myxomatous transformation, like fibrosis, appear to be a nonspecific tissue reaction to a variety of etiological factors (193,278). More extensive and severe degrees are associated with disruption of the valve, encroachment of the spongiosa into the fibrosa and the clinical syndrome of the idiopathic MVP ranging from the "silent" form, to isolated click, and to severe mitral regurgitation (175,306,336).

MISCELLANEOUS PATHOLOGICAL FINDINGS

Superficial fibrinous deposit over cracks in the endothelial surface (278) and thrombi in the acute angle between the prolapsed posterior leaflets and atrial wall (380) have been noted in valves showing myxomatous transformation. Endothelial denudation of the atrial aspect of involved leaflets has been observed with deposits of fibrin upon the denuded surface (150). Calcification of the posterior mitral leaflets involved by myxomatous change has been reported (150). It begins at the basal aspect of the leaflet and should not be confused with calcification of the mitral ring. In one of our patients, the posterior leaflet was heavily calcified and retracted (175) and in a second patient, one scallop of the posterior leaflet was calcified. Pulmonary emphysema and/or fibrosis were described in eight of 22 cases of myxomatous valves (150).

Chapter 4

Etiology

Two main theories have been advanced to explain the etiology of this syndrome. The first stresses mitral valve abnormality and the second myocardial involvement as demonstrated by left ventriculography and hemodynamic studies.

VALVULAR THEORY

Proponents of this theory hold that myxomatous transformation of the mitral valve is the underlying mechanism responsible for the idiopathic MVP syndrome. The loss of the collagenous supporting structure allows stretching of the cusps by the ventricular pressure and results in redundant and prolapsed leaflets. The valvular theory provides an explanation for the various manifestations of the click syndrome. The chest pain is ascribed to excessive traction on the papillary muscle by the chordae tendineae attached to a voluminous billowing leaflet that overshoots the other leaflet and lacks, therefore, its support (71,169,175,263,264). The loss of the "keystone effect" leads to disengagement of the leaflets with excessive tension on the papillary muscles and interference with their tenuous blood supply (73,276). Electrocardiographic changes and the ventricular arrhythmias are secondary to papillary muscle and endocardial ischemia and subsequent fibrosis. In experimental preparation (73,185), papillary muscle stretching has been shown to reduce propagation of action potential and to excite local pacemaker activity. Arrhythmias may also originate from the abnormally tensed mitral leaflets that contain muscle fibers capable of developing diastolic depolarization (389). Triggered activity in cardiac muscle fibers of the simian mitral valve was demonstrated (388). Sudden death is believed to be arrhythmic in origin. The click that coincides with maximal prolapse (85) is probably due to "sudden tensing of the everted valve leaflets," the "snapping of a sail phenomenon" (221) or to sudden deceleration of a mass of blood with resultant vibrations involving the heart chambers, valves, and contents (82). The late systolic murmur is attributed to the initially competent valve becoming incompetent as prolapse develops (85,357) and the pansystolic murmur to severe prolapse causing early separation of the leaflets. Response of the click and murmur to various maneuvers is explained by changes in left ventricular volume (175). The sharp systolic retraction observed on the apex cardiogram is ascribed to abnormal tension on the papillary muscle resulting in the base of this structure being drawn inward (276,343). The indentation along the inferior border of the left ventriculogram (148) may be due to the same mechanism (e.g., ventricular buckling) (73). Cobbs and King (72,73) reported a case of MVP with "abnormal inward motion at the site of the papillary muscle." Mitral valve replacement was carried out for intractable ventricular arrhythmias and one episode of ventricular fibrillation. Postoperatively, the left ventriculogram promptly returned to almost normal. This interesting case adds further support to the valvular theory and disproves theories postulating an abnormal contraction ring as a primary myocardial disorder responsible for the prolapse (322). The same authors have recently reported three other cases with the same regression of inward left ventricular motion after mitral valve replacement (148).

The pathologic basis of the valvular theory was described in detail in Chap. 3. This theory has been confirmed by the finding of myxomatous and redundant mitral valve cusps in 26 patients with midsystolic clicks. To my knowledge, these 26 cases represent the only available adequate pathological studies in patients with nonejection clicks and their importance lies in the demonstration of redundant myxomatous cusps in each instance when a click had been heard. It is of interest that three of these patients, females aged 6, 13 and 24 respectively, had no symptoms of cardiac dysfunction and died of cancer (19,304). The pathological evidence is much more extensive in patients who have pansystolic murmurs and mitral insufficiency as a complication of the advanced form of myxomatous degeneration, "the floppy valve." Furthermore normal mitral cusps have not been demonstrated at surgery or at autopsy in patients known to have had nonejection clicks.

Critique of the Valvular Theory

The sparcity of morphological data is due to the good prognosis of most patients with the click syndrome. More clinical morphologic correlations are needed before concluding that myxomatous deformed leaflets or scallops are the underlying pathological findings in all patients who have a "silent" MVP or a nonejection click with or without a murmur.

MYOCARDIAL THEORY

This theory is based primarily on angiographic and hemodynamic correlations. Recently histological support has been provided in an abstract authored by the Stanford group (199). Although some workers have implicated coronary artery disease (11,12,66,288,350), most advocates of the myocardial theory have postulated a segmental cardiomyopathy unrelated to this disease. They ascribe chest pain, dyspnea, arrhythmia and the ECG changes to primary myocardial involvement. Their disparate findings are as follows (179) (Table 4.1).

TABLE 4.1. *Arguments invoked by proponents of the myocardial theory*

---

1. Abnormal systolic protrusion of the inferior aspect of the LV
2. Noncontraction or late systolic expansion of the inflow tract of the LV
3. Asynergy of LV
4. Hemodynamic disturbances
5. Myocardial lactate abnormalities
6. Echocardiographic findings
7. Interstitial fibrosis on right ventricular biopsy

---

1. Abnormal systolic protrusion of the inferior wall of the left ventricle (148) which results in elevation of the papillary muscles. The chordae tendineae become slack allowing the posterior leaflet to balloon into the left atrium.

2. Noncontraction or late systolic expansion of the inflow tract of the left ventricle with significant reduction in the extent and mean velocity of fiber shortening in this segment (222). Congenital absence of the atrioventricular groove branch of the left coronary artery reported by one group in 17 of 19 patients with MVP (137), was felt to be responsible for this segmental myocardial dysfunction.

3. Left ventricular assynergy. Gooch et al. (144) described assynergistic contraction or relaxation in 17 of their patients: 16 had an anterior convex bulging during late systole or early diastole and 8 of these had systolic bulging of the inferoposterior wall. One patient had apical akinesia. The same group (322) had subsequently described five types of abnormal left ventricular systolic contraction patterns:

a. "Ballerina foot" pattern (vigorous posteromedial contraction with anterior convexity)

b. "Hourglass" pattern (vigorous ringlike contraction involving the middle portion of the left ventricle)

c. Inadequate shortening of the long axis

d. Posterior akinesia

e. Pattern of cavity obliteration.

4. Hemodynamic disturbances. I described a constrictive pattern of the left ventricular pressure curves in five of my original 32 cases (169). In the absence of severe mitral regurgitation, hemodynamic studies have generally shown no abnormalities (175,322). However, Gulotta et al. (149) reported, in 20 of their 26 patients, left ventricular dysfunction documented by either elevated left ventricular end-diastolic pressure, low resting cardiac index, or inappropriate rise in cardiac index during exercise.

5. Abnormal myocardial metabolic studies: Myocardial lactate abnormalities have been described in this syndrome both at rest and during pacing

(111,194,261,270). These abnormalities were felt to be due either to "small vessel disease" or to the abnormal cellular metabolism of cardiomyopathy (270).

6. Echocardiographic findings: Mathey et al. (236) demonstrated a reduction in max V_{cf} during the preprolapse period. They felt that this reduction in left ventricular contractility which was noted in the preprolapse period was, therefore, unrelated to a direct mechanical effect of the prolapse itself.

7. Mild to moderate interstitial fibrosis in right ventricular biopsy specimen (158).

Critique of the Myocardial Theory

Disparate angiographic features were described by various authors ranging from akinesia (222) to hypercontractility (148,170,322), from hypokinesis of the inferior wall (222) to abnormal systolic protrusion of the same wall (148) and from assynergy of the anterior wall with systolic bulging (144,149) to vigorous contraction involving the same area (322). To confuse the picture further, other workers (96) reported a normal contracting pattern in 72% of their patients. Therefore, the contraction pattern shows a broad variation that argues against its primary role in determining the abnormal valve motion (283). To explain these contradictory findings disparate causes of the same syndrome have to be postulated, thus prompting an explanation for these discrepancies (179). The angiographic abnormalities may be factitial and due to the effect of premature ventricular contractions induced during the injection of dye (112). Eber et al. (112) described assynergy resulting from premature ventricular contractions and ventricular tachycardia with apically stimulated left ventricular beats producing an "hourglass" type of contraction and basal stimulation producing inversed "teardrop" pattern; they warned against the hazards of misinterpretation of left ventricular contraction pattern if the beats originate ectopically during ventriculography. The assynergistic effect of PVCs was well documented in one of our patients who underwent two angiographic studies 4 years apart: marked assynergy associated with a run of premature ventricular contractions was noted during the first study but not during the second study, which was free of arrhythmias (179). Even if genuine, the abnormalities of the left ventricular contraction do not necessarily indicate a primary myocardial disease. Rigidity of various segments of the left ventricle, particularly near the inflow tract, may be due to fibrotic friction lesions (317). Traction on the posterior papillary muscle with ventricular buckling may explain the indentation along the inferior left ventricular wall (73,175). Buckling of both papillary muscle sites and bulky papillary muscles would explain the "ballerina foot" and the "hourglass" or "cavity obliteration" patterns (73). Excessive contractility may be due to aneurysmal ballooning of the easily distensible cusps reducing the volume of blood encompassed by the muscular element (179) and, therefore, unloading the left ventricle (264). Thus MVP per se mimics the effect of mitral insufficiency decreasing left ventricular afterload and increasing the velocity and extent of fiber shortening (170). The sum of all these factors related to the prolapsed redundant leaflets may result in a spectrum of angiographic manifestations without the need to postulate focal myocardiopathy. Moreover, abundant observations have established the primacy of mitral prolapse in patients without detectable abnormalities of left ventricular contractility (108).

The hemodynamic disturbances, when present, may be due to associated mitral regurgitation or to endocardial, subendocardial, and papillary muscle ischemia and fibrosis. Decreased left ventricular compliance resulting from these endocardial and subendocardial changes would explain the constrictive pattern.

The abnormal lactate metabolism both at rest and after pacing may be due to papillary muscle ischemia secondary to traction by the prolapsed leaflets. The increased heart rate induced by pacing reduces left ventricular volume, inducing, therefore, more prolapse, more traction, and more ischemia.

A major argument against the myocardial theory is the absence of clicks and echocardiographic evidence of MVP in primary and secondary myocardial disease. Involvement of the papillary muscle has been described in sarcoidosis and amyloidosis but auscultatory or echocardiographic evidence of MVP have not been reported in these diseases. To my knowledge, only two cases of late systolic click in primary cardiomyopathy have been reported (250), raising the question of coincidental occurrence of two common entities. In my series, I observed the development of severe cardiomyopathy in a young woman who presented with a midsystolic click and left bundle branch block at age 32, and who developed an additional late systolic murmur at age 37. At age 43, she was seen in severe heart failure and massive cardiomegaly was noted; a pansystolic murmur was heard and minimal mitral regurgitation and markedly reduced ejection fraction were observed on left ventriculography (Fig. 4.1).

In hypertrophic subaortic stenosis, I described angiographic prolapse due to a reduced left ventricular cavity (170) and termed it "secondary ballooning"; however, my associates and I have not heard nonejection clicks in more than 100 patients with this disease. Others (365) reported clicks in a handful of cases, and this finding may represent the casual occurrence of two common diseases in the same individual. These clicks may also be related to a sudden halting of the systolic anterior motion of the anterior leaflet as shown by Sze and Shah (356) in their echophonocardiographic studies. To the best of my knowledge, echocardiographic prolapse of the posterior leaflet has never been shown in hypertrophic subaortic stenosis. However, the

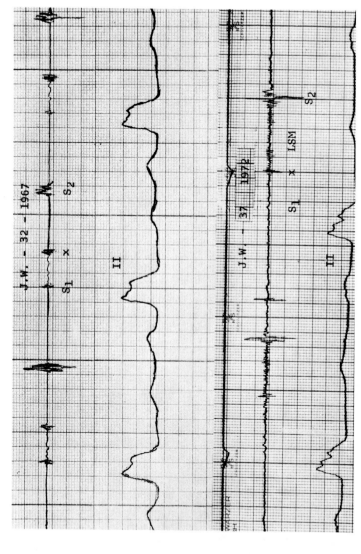

FIG. 4.1. Case 88. Apex phonocardiogram of a 32-year-old woman who developed cardiomyopathy during an 11-year follow-up. Coronary arteriogram was normal. A. Early to midsystolic click (×) and left bundle branch block at age 32. B. Midsystolic click (×) and late systolic murmur (LSM) at age 37. An isolated pansystolic murmur was heard at age 43. (See text).

association between MVP and assymetric septal hypertrophy was reported in 16 out of 190 consecutive cases of MVP proven by echocardiography (65). The significance of this observation is not clear. Further correlation is needed, particularly in view of the recent emphasis on the nonspecific nature of assymetric septal hypertrophy as noted on echocardiography.

The mild to moderate interstitial fibrosis noted by the Stanford group (158) on right ventricular biopsy provides a histological support for the myocardial theory. However, these findings may be secondary to associated tricuspid prolapse and right ventricular friction lesions that were not ruled out in their studies. Other pathologists (305,336) did not note myocardial abnormalities and the Stanford group itself reported normal endomyocardial biopsy in three patients with click syndrome, angina, and a normal coronary arteriogram (200).

RELATION BETWEEN CORONARY ARTERY DISEASE AND THE MITRAL VALVE PROLAPSE–CLICK SYNDROME

Papillary muscle dysfunction resulting from coronary artery disease has been held by some workers (11,12,19,66,83,221,288,350,369) to be responsible for this syndrome. In a few reported cases (19,67,83,350) a non-ejection click was heard in patients with proven coronary artery disease and occasionally, the echocardiogram was reported as being diagnostic of MVP (288). However, in most of these reports, only a late systolic murmur was heard or MVP was only noted on left ventriculography. In one case (83), reported to illustrate the causal relationship between coronary artery disease and MVP, a click was not heard before or after the first myocardial infarction, and an angiographic study in the *RAO position* was reported as showing no MVP; occlusion of the left anterior descending coronary artery was noted. Following a second infarction, 6 months later, a click and a late systolic murmur were heard and a repeat study demonstrated occlusion of the left circumflex and MVP i:, the *LAO position*. I believe that the first cine left ventriculogram in the RAO position did show prolapse of the posteromedial scallop of the posterior leaflet but the second study was more diagnostic of MVP. Left ventriculograms in two views should not be compared because in some patients the LAO view may be more diagnostic of MVP and vice versa. It is also possible that the click was evanescent and was only heard after the second infarction.

Steelman et al. (350) reported 15 instances of click-murmur in 700 patients with coronary artery disease.

Pathological correlations in patients with coronary artery disease and MVP was reported in only one patient with known click (67) and in seven patients with either late systolic murmur or angiographic evidence of MVP (10,67,369). No redundancy or myxomatous degeneration was reported in these cases.

Experimentally, angiographic MVP was induced in the dog (5 out of 10 cases) following coronary artery occlusion (117).

Critique of the Coronary Theory

In discussing the relationship of coronary artery disease and mitral valve prolapse–click syndrome, emphasis should be placed on the prevalence of these two diseases leading to their casual occurrence in the same patients (172,174,175,179). As pointed out by Devereux et al. (108) the finding of Steelman et al. (350) of 15 instances of click-murmur in a population of 700 patients with coronary artery disease yields a prevalence of 2%. This is close to the prevalence of MVP in the general population. The rare occurrence of a click in patients with proven coronary artery disease on one hand and the demonstration of normal coronary arteriogram in about 98% of patients known to have a click on the otherhand confirm a casual rather than a causal relationship of these two common entities. The following points are essential to this discussion:

1. Late systolic murmurs can undoubtedly be due to papillary muscle dysfunction (92,102,155) but it must be proved that midsystolic clicks, the auscultatory hallmark of idiopathic MVP can be caused by this disorder. This association between click and papillary muscle dysfunction is not evident in three comprehensive reviews of papillary muscle dysfunction (92,102,155). Burch et al. (47) state: "Late systolic clicks have to the present time, not been observed as a feature of the papillary muscle dysfunction syndrome secondary to ischemic heart disease." (Table 4.2).

2. In acute myocardial infarction, which is often associated with the murmur of papillary muscle dysfunction (155), the occurrence of non-ejection clicks is most uncommon. Over the years, I have asked various medical audiences about their observations as to the occurrence de novo of clicks in the coronary care unit and I have been impressed by its almost total absence. In a 3-year prospective study in our coronary care unit, which admits about 700 patients annually, we have observed no patients who developed clicks de novo in the course of acute myocardial infarction (175). Fourth heart sounds and systolic murmurs but not clicks are the most common auscultatory findings in the coronary care unit. If coronary artery disease were a cause of the mitral valve prolapse–click syndrome, one would have expected the click to be a common auscultatory finding in coronary care units.

The few cases of de novo occurrence of clicks in acute myocardial infarction (67,83) may be due to the known evanescent nature of these clicks. Another explanation may be that the critical left ventricular volume at which the click occurs (242) may not have been reached in the initial stages of acute myocardial infarction because of depressed ejection fraction. As the ejection fraction increases in the course of hospitalization, a previously heard

TABLE 4.2. *Idiopathic MVP and coronary artery disease: Common and distinguishing features*

	Redundant myxomatous mitral cusps	Click	Late systolic or pansystolic murmurs	Coronary arteries	Angiographic prolapse	Echocardiographic prolapse
Idiopathic Mitral Valve Prolapse	Yes	Yes	Yes	Normal	Yes	Yes
Papillary muscle dysfunction in coronary artery disease	No	No	Yes	Obstructive lesions	Yes	No

click that was absent on admission to the coronary care unit may become audible again. If these patients are seen for the first time during their hospitalization for acute myocardial infarction, one may mistakenly, therefore, label the click as a new finding and attribute it to the myocardial infarction.

3. A distinction should be made between the click and the angiographic

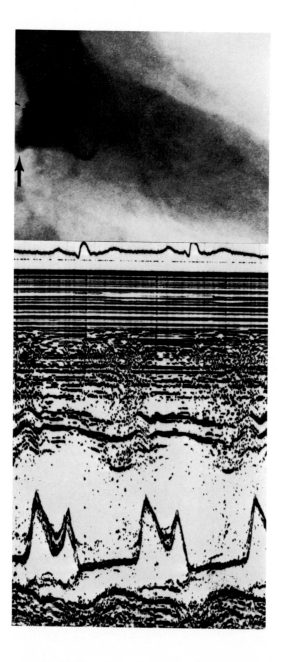

FIG. 4.2. Angiographic prolapse involving the middle (upper arrow) and the posteromedial (lower arrow) scallops of the posterior leaflet in a patient with proven coronary artery disease and no click or murmur (angiographic-auscultatory discordance). The echocardiogram reveals no prolapse (angiographic–echocardiographic discordance).

evidence of MVP. Prolapse of the leaflets, which are not anchored during ejection by contraction of the ischemic or infarcted papillary muscles, is the underlying mechanism of papillary muscle dysfunction in coronary artery disease. A spectrum of clinical and angiographic manifestations is noted ranging from the "silent" form which can only be detected by angiography to the regurgitant form which is associated with auscultatory and angiographic evidence of mitral regurgitation. My angiographic observations lead me to concur with those who have reported a high prevalence of angiographic prolapse in ischemic heart disease in the absence of mitral regurgitation (12,288,340,369) (Figs. 4.2 and 4.3). In one series (12) ventriculography following coronary artery bypass surgery in two patients showed improved contraction and disappearance of previously visualized leaflet prolapse. Yet, except for a rare case which is compatible with casual occurrence, clicks were not heard in these patients (2,179). I have termed the paradoxical occurrence of angiographic MVP in patients with coronary artery disease in the absence of a click "angiographic–auscultatory discordance" (182) (Table 4.1). I postulate that a prerequisite for the production of a click is the presence of abnormal and redundant mitral cusps as noted in idiopathic MVP, but not in coronary artery disease with angiographic prolapse.

4. In our experience and in that of others (280,340) MVP is not observed

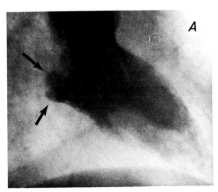
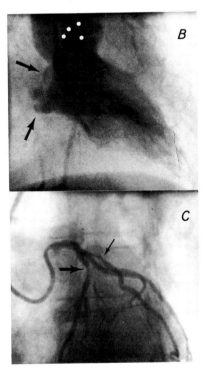

FIG. 4.3. A and B. Angiographic prolapse involving the 3 scallops of the posterior leaflets (arrows) in a 52-year-old woman with coronary artery disease, and no auscultatory (angiographic-auscultatory discordance) or echocardiographic (angiographic–echocardiographic discordance) abnormalities. C. Selective left coronary arteriogram in a 30° LAO view shows severe proximal stenosis of the anterior descending artery and of its diagonal branch (left arrow) and moderately severe stenosis of the left marginal circumflex (right arrow). The anterolateral scallop of the posterior leaflet is outlined by dots (B).

TABLE 4.3. *The left circumflex arterial circulation in 45 patients with mitral valve prolapse*

A. A-V groove branch present		37
1. Predominant right coronary circulation	25	
2. Predominant left coronary circulation	7	
3. Balanced coronary circulation	5	
B. A-V groove branch absent		8
1. Large posterolateral branch of right coronary artery	7	
2. Small posterolateral branch of right coronary artery	1	

by echocardiography in patients with ischemic papillary muscle dysfunction despite the angiographic evidence of prolapse in these patients (Table 4.2). I have no explanation for this intriguing echocardiographic–angiographic discordance in coronary artery disease. This discordance is not evident in the idiopathic mitral valve prolapse–click syndrome in which echocardiography is positive in about 80 to 90% of patients. It is possible that echocardiography can detect MVP only if the cusps are redundant and voluminous.

5. Since coronary artery disease does not induce myxomatous transformation of the mitral valve, the demonstration of a midsystolic click and of a positive echo in patients with coronary artery disease and a nonmyxomatous mitral valve would be the only convincing evidence that could causally link these two entities (175). Only one such case of midsystolic click, coronary artery disease and normal valve at autopsy has been reported in a letter to the editor (67).

Coronary Artery Distribution in Patients with Prolapse of the Mitral Valve

As mentioned above, Gentzler et al. (137) reported congenital absence of the atrioventricular groove branch of the left circumflex coronary artery. Review of the coronary arteriograms in 45 of our patients revealed this finding in only eight patients. Seven of these eight patients had a large posterolateral branch of the right coronary artery to compensate for this absence which is probably a normal variant (Table 4.3). Others (140,369) have also shown a normal coronary artery distribution in patients with mitral prolapse.

Primary Versus Secondary MVP

The concept of idiopathic or primary prolapse versus secondary prolapse is needed to elucidate the association of coronary artery disease, hypertrophic subaortic stenosis, etc. with mitral valve prolapse. I presented this concept in 1971 (170) in an attempt to differentiate the myxomatous MVP that I termed primary ballooning from the angiographic prolapse of the posterior leaflet found in hypertrophic subaortic stenosis that I termed secondary. Others (2,10,84,264) adopted the same classification and applied it to other etiologies of MVP. On the basis of the available auscultatory pathologic correlations in the 26 cases with clicks mentioned above, I believe that it is reasonable to state that the finding of a nonejection click is indicative of primary myxomatous mitral valve prolapse. In 80 to 90% of these patients, echocardiography and left ventricular angiography would demonstrate diagnostic evidence of prolapse. A typical clinical and electrocardiographic syndrome may be associated with the click in these patients.

Secondary MVP is essentially an angiographic finding. In these patients, clicks are not heard, the echo shows no prolapse and the clinical picture, morbidity and mortality are "related to the underlying disease process rather than to the mitral valve dysfunction" (84). The major impact of the concept of secondary prolapse is on the angiographic diagnosis. To those championing a causal relationship of coronary artery disease and MVP, one should admit that angiographically this is true but pathologically, clinically, echocardiographically, and prognostically the dissociation is clearcut. Angiographic prolapse is a nonspecific finding and its demonstration in a patient with coronary artery disease can be considered as an incidental occurrence with no known significance except that it probably indicates papillary muscle dysfunction. In coronary artery disease, the finding of MVP on left ventriculography does not warrant the diagnosis of an additional disease or syndrome (e.g., idiopathic mitral valve prolapse) because in these patients the mitral valve does not show myxomatous transformation, no click is heard, and the echocardiogram is negative for MVP. The clinical picture is not affected by the finding of angiographic MVP except when a click is heard and the echocardiogram is positive in which case the two diseases may be coexisting and the chest pain may be caused by either one (Fig. 12.25).

In the presence of a left ventriculogram diagnostic of MVP, the demonstration of coronary artery disease probably indicates that the angiographic finding is related to it and has no special significance. However, if a click is heard or the echocardiogram is diagnostic of MVP, then one is dealing with two common diseases occurring independently in the same patient.

Angiocardiographers, whose caseloads are primarily made up of patients with coronary artery disease, detect MVP so often that they tend to call it a normal variant and to ignore, its significance in young patients with atypical chest pain and normal coronary arteriograms.

Unfortunately, several articles (12,288,369) dealing with coronary artery disease and MVP have not stressed that their findings were purely angiographic and that the syndrome of MVP-click syndrome shares only angiographic features with coronary artery disease. These angiographic articles and others that reported a probable casual association between click and coronary artery disease have created the impression in the literature of a causal linking between coronary artery disease and the idiopathic click syndrome (179). The click has been described by some workers as a clinical clue in coronary artery disease (81).

It is essential to stress that any relationship between coronary artery disease and nonejection clicks is casual and that coronary artery disease and idiopathic click syndrome share only the angiographic features the same way coronary artery disease and cardiomyopathy share several electrocardiographic features but not the same etiology, the same clinical features and the same coronary artery anatomy.

I do not wish to detract from the value of left ventriculography in the diagnosis of MVP, particularly in the auscultatory silent form (178). In this clinical form, however, coronary artery disease is not present, the clinical and echocardiographic features are similar to the typical click syndrome, and the echocardiogram is often diagnostic.

Coronary Artery Spasm and Small Coronary Artery Vessel Disease in MVP

Four young patients with MVP (three with clicks that were intermittent in two and only one with left ventricular angiogram diagnostic of MVP) who presented with evidence of acute myocardial infarction were reported by Chesler et al. (70). Because the coronary arteriogram was normal and the electrocardiogram showed pronounced elevation of S-T segment, these authors postulated spasm of normal coronary arteries as the operative factor. They advocated scrutiny of those cases of ischemic heart disease with normal coronary arteriogram to establish whether there is in fact a causal relationship with MVP. The spasm was felt to be a reflex response to billowing of the posterior leaflet or to the injured papillary muscle. Myers et al. (257) have reported MVP in seven out of eight patients with catheter induced spasm and normal coronary arteriogram. Awdeh and Gholston (15), have demonstrated spasm of a prolonged segment of the right coronary artery in a 55-year-old women with a history of prolonged episodes of chest pain, midsystolic click and late systolic murmur on auscultation, prolapse of the posterior leaflet on left ventricular angiogram and a normal coronary arteriogram except for the transient spasm.

Chesler's et al.'s (70) cases are intriguing and would warrant further observation to rule out the possibility of a chance association between MVP and myocardial infarction with normal coronary arteriogram. In future studies, it is essential that the diagnosis of MVP be made on the basis of a click or if the diagnosis of MVP is made angiographically, the left ventriculogram should have been performed prior to the occurrence of myocardial infarction because the papillary muscle dysfunction resulting from myocardial infarction may be associated with angiographic prolapse, a nonspecific finding in this syndrome. As pointed out by Chesler et al. (70) the coronary arterial spasm postulated by them is seldom associated with acute myocardial infarction. Moreover, patients with Prinzmetal's angina have recurrent episodes of chest pain but this was not the case in three out of four of Chesler's patients who experience their first episode of chest pain when they developed their acute myocardial infarction.

A more attractive hypothesis to explain Chesler's cases is that of a coronary artery embolism originating from the prolapsed leaflets. Superficial fibrinous deposits have been noted on prolapsed leaflets (278,380). A similar embolic mechanism was postulated to explain TIA in MVP. Coronary embolism would explain the sudden onset of acute myocardial infarction in the absence of previous chest pain and in the presence of a normal coronary arteriogram.

Catheter induced spasm is a common angiographic occurrence and further correlation is needed to establish a causal relationship between it and MVP, a prevalent syndrome. Chances of casual occurrence are quite high.

A relationship between prolapsing mitral valve and angina with normal coronary arteriogram was postulated by Nakhjavan et al. (259). Indeed, many of these patients with this form of angina turn out to have idiopathic MVP and some, hypertrophic subaortic stenosis. Echocardiography is most helpful in the evaluation of these patients. In the syndrome of angina-like chest pain with normal coronary arteriogram, it is possible that the resulting papillary muscle dysfunction may cause angiographic MVP but would not be expected to result in a click or a positive echocardiogram.

Small coronary artery abnormalities that are felt by a few workers to be the underlying pathology in angina with normal coronary arteriogram were not noted on right ventricular biopsy in MVP (199).

In Marfan's syndrome, which is often associated with MVP (43) the extramural coronary arteries, in four of five cases studied, showed structural changes consistent with accumulation of acid mucopolysaccharides and a concomitant disrupt'˘r of the connective tissue elements resembling "cystic medial necrosis" (24). The intramural coronary arteries were unaffected. These abnormalities have not yet been reported in idiopathic MVP but should be actively sought.

CORONARY ARTERY DISEASE AND MITRAL VALVE PROLAPSE: AN OVERVIEW

The available evidence does not warrant, therefore, suspicion of coronary artery disease when a click is heard and supports the converse view (e.g., that the finding of a click in a patient with atypical chest pain and ST-T changes would favor idiopathic MVP rather than coronary artery disease as the underlying disorder). However, coronary arteriography is warranted in such patients if the clinical picture (risk factors, age, exertional chest pain) suggests additional coronary artery disease.

The evidence that I have presented would also warrant the following conclusions:

1. In coronary artery disease with or without mitral regurgitation, left ventriculography may reveal mitral valve prolapse that is indistinguishable from the classic angiographic picture of prolapse in a young woman with a normal coronary arteriogram, a click and a diagnostic echocardiogram. Papillary muscle dysfunction is probably responsible for the angiographic prolapse in coronary artery disease. MVP in patients with coronary artery disease represents an intermediate stage before clinically apparent mitral regurgitation develops (12).

2. Nonejection clicks are not caused by coronary artery disease. When heard in patients with coronary artery disease, they represent a casual finding resulting from the coexistence of two prevalent entities.

3. The echocardiogram in ischemic papillary muscle dysfunction does not reveal the typical picture of prolapse.

VENTRICULOVALVULAR DISPROPORTION IN MVP

In discussing the etiology of MVP, Criley and Kissel (84) have postulated an anatomical or functional ventriculovalvular disproportion in which either the valve is "too big" for the ventricle or the ventricle is "too small" for the valve during the course of ventricular systole. Cheng (68) has advanced a similar theory in which he postulated a small left ventricular cavity in young women, in pectus excavatum, in atrial septal defect etc. to explain MVP. Despite their general appeal, these theories lack pathological confirmation. No cases of click and/or diagnostic echo have been reported with a normal nonmyxomatous mitral valve at surgery or autopsy. This theory may explain angiographic prolapse but not the total clinical picture.

MVP AND THE MARFAN SYNDROME

Myxomatous transformation has been described in Erdheim's cystic medial necrosis of the aorta and in the ascending aorta and mitral valve in Marfan's syndrome (175). Pronounced interchordal "hooding" and "overshooting" of mitral leaflets have also been described in Marfan's syndrome (114). Brown et al. (43) found an echocardiographic MVP prevalence of 91% and a murmur of mitral regurgitation and/or systolic clicks in 46% of 35 patients with Marfan's syndrome. MVP was demonstrated by echocardiography in 33% (13 out of 40) of first degree relatives of 19 patients with Marfan's syndrome (271). Of the 13 relatives with echocardiographic evidence of MVP, only six had either midsystolic click or a murmur of mitral regurgitation. However, oculoskeletal stigmata of Marfan's syndrome have been infrequent in large series of idiopathic MVP, being present in only four of our patients. Despite the absence of these stigmata, Read et al. (297)

ascribed myxomatous transformation of the mitral valve to a forme fruste of Marfan's syndrome. I believe that this conclusion, which is based on insufficient evidence, is not warranted because despite the high prevalence of MVP in Marfan's syndrome, there is a rare occurrence of Marfan's syndrome in idiopathic MVP. By analogy, dissecting aneurysm is a common complication of Marfan's syndrome but since there are other etiologies for dissection, there is no justification to label all dissections as a complication of a forme fruste of Marfan's syndrome. It is worth noting that dissecting aneurysm is an unheard of complication of idiopathic MVP, except as a complication of the application of aortic clamp to the ascending aorta during cardiopulmonary bypass in patients with "floppy" mitral valve (244).

MVP AND RHEUMATIC HEART DISEASE

Barlow and associates (19) emphasized the etiological relationship between rheumatic fever and the click syndrome on the basis of frequent association of these diseases in their series. Steinfeld et al. (352) have also reported this association; however, most of their patients had isolated late systolic murmur, a nonspecific finding, and only four of their 34 patients had clicks. The association of rheumatic mitral insufficiency and the ubiquitous nonejection click in such a small number of patients could be casual and does not warrant a causal correlation. In most reported series, rheumatic heart disease as defined by historical, clinical or pathological criteria was strikingly absent (175). In our series, only three patients related a history of rheumatic fever. It is possible that in South Africa the high prevalence of rheumatic fever in black children would explain the casual association of two common entities (e.g., rheumatic heart disease and idiopathic MVP).

The rheumatic process causes scarring, retraction, and commissural fusion rather than the characteristic redundancy and prolapse of myxomatous transformation (77,85,150,279). Guthrie and Edwards (150) described well the histological distinction between the rheumatic and myxomatous process even when secondary fibrotic changes in the latter yield a picture resembling superficially the rheumatic process. They showed that in the rheumatic valve there is fibrosis of the entire substance of the leaflet with loss of distinction of one layer from another. In contrast in the myxomatous valve with the use of special stains, the specific layers of the leaflet are identifiable.

I have noted angiographic MVP in some patients with proven mitral stenosis, in the absence of a click or echocardiographic evidence of MVP. The angiographic finding may be nonspecific (340); however its significance should be established in future studies by echocardiographic and pathological correlations. Recently, MVP associated with rheumatic mitral stenosis was reported in nine patients (375,380). All four patients in one study (375) had histories of rheumatic fever and echocardiograms diagnostic of both mitral stenosis and MVP. However none of these patients had a non-ejection click. The commissural fusion may have interfered, in an unknown fashion, with the mechanism of production of the click. Three of these patients underwent cine ventriculography that confirmed the presence of mitral stenosis and showed systolic prolapse and excessive scalloping of the mitral valve. Two patients underwent mitral valve surgery that revealed commissural fusion, large redundant leaflets and myxomatous degeneration. It is likely, as the authors stated that "the relationship between these two disease in the present cases is coincidental."

However, it is possible that mitral stenosis may result from altered flow across a myxomatous redundant valve leading to cusp thickening and rigidity and eventually to commissural fusion. A similar mechanism has been invoked to explain the development of aortic stenosis on rheumatic valvulitis or on congenital deformity. The patients with combined MVP and mitral stenosis should be investigated with this concept in mind. Long term followup of MVP patients without a history of rheumatic fever for the development of mitral stenosis should provide an answer to this question.

NATURE OF THE MYXOMATOUS PROCESS

The myxomatous or myxoid stroma is a part of the normal valve. Minimal increase in this stroma is commonly found in diseased valves as a nonspecific reaction similar to fibrosis. When severe, this process becomes disruptive and associated with a typical pathological and a clinical picture of idiopathic MVP. In a few reported series, this process was genetically determined, but in most cases it constitutes a nonspecific reaction to various factors and possibly to the wear and tear of valvular movement.

Abnormalities of connective tissue similar to myxomatous transformation have been described in experimental lathyrism (175). The latter results from excessive ingestion of peas of the genus lathyrus which contains beta-amino-proprionitrile. The occurrence of these connective tissues abnormalities in response to ingestion of particular chemicals raises the possibility that extraneous chemical agents may be responsible for human myxomatous mitral transformation.

The myxomatous process is most often seen in the elderly, but "this fact is more an expression of the long natural history than an indication that aging itself is the etiological factor." (279). The low incidence of advanced myxomatous degeneration in the elderly indicates that this degeneration is not an involutionary process and the slight increase with aging is merely an expression of the increasing incidence of disease process generally (279).

The myxomatous mitral transformation is probably an end result of local factors rather than a primary defect in mucopolysaccharide metabolism (337). However, the frequent occurrence of thoracic skeletal abnormalities

(38,318) and of pulmonary emphysema (150,400) would suggest a generalized connective tissue disorder.

It is essential, therefore, to concentrate future investigations on the nature and cause of the myxomatous process and to seek possible anomalies of polysaccharides metabolism. It is my contention that further research into the nature of this process is to quote Sutton's law, "where the money is" (179).

Chapter 5

Symptomatology

Symptomatology in idiopathic MVP is variable and includes chest pain, lightheadedness, dyspnea, fatigue, and palpitations (Table 5.1). Only 20 of our first 100 patients were free of these symptoms (175) as were only 25% of Hancock and Cohn's 40 patients (154) and 13% of Malcolm et al.'s 85 patients (231). These figures for patients referred to a cardiology service do not give a true picture of the prevalence of symptoms in an unscreened population with idiopathic MVP. Most of the patients evaluated in cardiology services are referred because of symptoms; chest pain was the presenting symptom in 46% and dyspnea in 9% of 40 patients in one series (231). The true prevalence of symptoms in idiopathic MVP will have to be established from large surveys of healthy populations screened by auscultation and/or echocardiography for MVP. Unfortunately, these surveys have concentrated on the asymptomatic normal (36,45), eliminating therefore patients whose symptoms may have been due to MVP. It is evident from the review of reported series that further studies are required to determine the true prevalence of symptoms of idiopathic MVP and that it is definitely below the 80% figure reported by referral cardiology centers. Some internists (285) feel that the overwhelming majority of patients with classic MVP seen in the practice of internal medicine do not have cardiovascular symptoms but are discovered during a routine examination or an examination for an unrelated condition. A prospective study by internists is needed to substantiate this impression.

Symptoms in MVP are usually mild but occasionally they are severe and incapacitating, precipitating extensive cardiac evaluation, emergency room visits, or coronary care unit admissions (283).

TABLE 5.1. Symptoms in idiopathic mvp

Chest pain	Syncope
Dyspnea	Palpitations
Fatigue	Transient ischemic attacks
Dizziness	Psychiatric manifestations

CHEST PAIN

Chest pain is the most common and potentially most disabling symptom in idiopathic MVP (18,108,154,175,215,220,231,264,380). It was reported by 61% of our patients (175) and was unrelated to activity in 83%, exertional in 8%, and occurred both at rest and on activity in 9%. The chest pain is less related to specific effort than to accumulation of fatigue (71). In most patients (215) it is not relieved by nitrates. It is usually "ill defined," left precordial, sharp, and either fleeting or lasting several hours" (175) or sometimes several weeks (231). The pain may disappear dramatically for a period of time and recur unexpectedly (71,108). In a few patients, despite a normal coronary arteriogram, exercise-induced chest pain, indistinguishable from angina, occurs (19,161,215). Some of these patients are hospitalized with suspected myocardial infarction. In a few patients (as in two of ours) the chest pain may mimic the mode of presentation of unstable angina because of its duration and the association of ECG abnormalities, and requires coronary arteriography to rule out coronary artery disease.

In six of our patients with severe chest pain, the erroneous diagnosis of acute pericarditis was made by the admitting internist or pediatrician, who had mistaken multiple clicks and precordial honks for the systolic component of a pericardial friction rub.

In a study by Lewinter et al. (220) chest pain was induced by phenylephrine infusion. However, the use of phenylephrine has given confusing results to others, as it failed to duplicate the pain in patients with severe prolapse and elicited discomfort when angiographic evidence of MVP was absent or minimal (73).

Idiopathic MVP, a prevalent syndrome, is probably a more common cause of chest pain than other etiologies that are postulated to explain pain in the absence of coronary artery disease (175).

Pathogenesis of Chest Pain in MVP

The pathogenesis of chest pain in this syndrome remains unknown. It has been ascribed to ischemia resulting from excessive traction of the prolapsed leaflets and their chordae on the papillary muscles (169,175,263,276). Normally the leaflets tightly coapt, bearing by their mutual support most of the systolic left ventricular pressure; when they fail to coapt, the full systolic thrust is placed upon the chordae, leading to excessive tugging on the papillary muscles. This traction interferes with the tenuous and precarious blood supply of the papillary muscle. Local coronary spasm due to mild focal trauma or papillary traction was postulated by Cobbs (71).

Basing their conclusion on the phenlyephrine test, Lewinter et al. attributed the chest pain to increased tension in "the areas at the base of the papillary muscles" (220). However, increase in left ventricular volume resulting from the phenylephrine-induced rise in blood pressure would be expected to decrease the severity of mitral prolapse and the resulting tension on the papillary muscle. It is not only difficult to reconcile these two opposing effects of phenylephrine (e.g., increase in wall tension and decrease in prolapse), but also other workers could not duplicate the phenylephrine results in their patients (73).

Compression of the left circumflex coronary artery in the atrioventricular groove by the prolapsed leaflet was postulated by Barlow et al. (33) but could not be confirmed by selective coronary arteriography (175).

Management of Chest Pain in MVP

The chest pain often responds to reassuring and convincing the patient that he is suffering from a benign disorder rather than from coronary artery disease. To stress the benign nature of the pain, the patient may be given a superficial explanation such as, "Some people have headaches, you have chestaches" (71). Propranolol is the drug of choice for relief of chest pain (19,175,215,339) because it (a) suppresses the excessive left ventricular contractility in this syndrome; (b) increases left ventricular volume, thus decreasing the prolapse; and (c) decreases the heart rate with resulting increase in the left ventricular volume, prevention of increased contractility, and thus reduction of the extent of prolapse. However, the beneficial effect of propranolol in chest pain was not evident in Winkle et al.'s (385) eight patients; chest pain was relieved in only two, unchanged in five, and became worse in one.

Unfortunately, patients with MVP seem to have less tolerance for propranolol than patients with angina pectoris. Even small dosage (e.g., 10 mg t.i.d. or q.i.d.) may be associated with increase in fatigue, a common symptom in this syndrome, and with development of mental depression. The usual dosage required for relief of chest pain is approximately 20 mg q.i.d.

Theoretically, nitrates should be contraindicated for the chest pain associated with this syndrome (264) because they reduce left ventricular volume and increase heart rate, both of which tend to increase the extent and duration of prolapse. In a few patients, however, chest pain responds to nitrates. O'Rourke and Crawford state, "Currently there is insufficient information on the use of nitrates in this syndrome to provide an accurate assessment" (264). I have recently been recommending the Trendelenburg position to some patients disabled by chest pain, hoping to increase venous return and left ventricular volume and thus to decrease the severity of prolapse. This position has been effective in the three patients who have used it for relief of pain. A few patients with disabling chest pain may have to be referred to "pain clinics."

Mitral valve replacement was carried out in one patient with intractable chest pain and resulted in relief of symptoms during a two year follow-up period (224). Cooley et al. (78) used a posterior annular collar prosthesis for surgical repair of MVP in eight patients with good subjective results. However, three of their patients had coronary artery disease. This series is too small and the results too preliminary to allow judgment on the value and effectiveness of this drastic approach for the relief of symptoms. In a subsequent abstract, the same group (395) reported on its experience with posterior annular collar prosthesis in 93 patients with mitral or tricuspid valve prolapse. Early mortality among patients undergoing insertion of the mitral C ring was 11.8%. Approximately two-thirds of these 93 patients underwent other cardiac surgical procedures. The indication for this operation is not clear in the abstract and this operation was probably used for relief of mitral and tricuspid regurgitation rather than for relief of various symptoms including chest pain. The authors state only that: "All surviving patients experienced a satisfactory clinical result with complete relief of mitral or tricuspid insufficiency with no murmurs of regurgitation audible following operation" (395).

DYSPNEA AND FATIGUE

Dyspnea and fatigue are often the presenting symptoms in this syndrome and were related by 60 of our first 100 patients (175). Dyspnea was present in 18 patients, fatigue in 22, and both in 20. Both symptoms were common in other series (18,154). In our series, there was equal distribution between mitral regurgitation and lack of mitral regurgitation in patients suffering from these symptoms, indicating, therefore, that there is no correlation between these symptoms and the presence of mitral regurgitation. There is poor correlation between these symptoms and treadmill exercise tolerance in these patients.

The pathogenesis of fatigue and dyspnea has not been elucidated. It is possible that in some patients they may be "psychoneurotic" in origin. Dyspnea may be due to hyperventilation (154). In some patients, dyspnea and fatigue may be iatrogenic due to impaired cardiovascular conditioning in patients whose activity has been restricted by their physician because of chest pain, heart murmur, or abnormal electrocardiogram. In pulmonary function studies carried out by our group there was no correlation between dyspnea and the increased residual volume noted in 63% of 20 patients with MVP and the reduced steady state diffusing capacity noted in 50% of the same group (400). No relationship was found between dyspnea and thoracic skeletal abnormalities.

I recently used amitriptyline (20 to 25 mg at bedtime) in three patients complaining of severe fatigue with excellent subjective response. The recent report of antiarrhythmic, quinidine-like effect of tricyclic antidepressants

(31) encouraged me to use this drug without fear of causing arrhythmias and with the hope of supressing them. Further study of the beneficial effect of tricyclic antidepressants on fatigue and on arrhythmias in this syndrome is needed before advocating their use.

LIGHTHEADEDNESS, DIZZINESS, AND SYNCOPE

These symptoms were related by approximately one-third of our patients (175). Four of these had experienced syncope. There was a relatively high incidence of syncope (six out of 12) in patients who died suddenly (384), suggesting a predictive value for syncope in sudden death. Wigle et al. (380) recorded seven instances of ventricular fibrillation as a cause of syncope in this syndrome; spontaneous defibrillation was observed in three of four patients with recurrent syncope. It is imperative, therefore, to obtain a 24-hr ambulatory monitoring of all patients with a history of syncope.

These symptoms often, but not always, are related to arrhythmias (384). In two of our cases, recurrent dizziness was not associated with any rhythm disturbance on ambulatory monitoring.

PALPITATIONS

Palpitations are frequently the presenting symptom in this syndrome (128,144,231) and were noted by 46% of our patients (175). They are often arrhythmic in origin and due to frequent premature ventricular beats, sinus tachycardia or paroxysmal supraventricular tachycardia, and so forth. Surprisingly, correlation between palpitations and arrhythmias is not always evident on 24-hr ambulatory monitoring: there were no changes in the patients' rhythm during three of eight palpitation episodes (384). I am able to confirm this observation. As will be pointed out later on, sudden onset of sinus tachycardia is often responsible for palpitations.

TRANSIENT ISCHEMIC ATTACKS

Transient ischemic attacks (TIAs) were recently reported in 12 patients with mitral valve prolapse and no evidence of infective endocarditis (21). All 12 patients had MVP proven by angiography, five were found to have midsystolic clicks, and eight had an echocardiogram indicative of MVP. Seven were men and five women, ranging in age from 18 to 67 with an average age of 38 years. The neurological picture was characterized by multiple attacks in eight, and a single attack in four. The more frequent episodes were typical of the abrupt onset of TIAs with early resolution. The attacks consisted of transient hemiparesis or major stroke in nine of 12 patients with unilateral sensory loss in four, dysarthria in three, aphasia in three, hemianopsia in three, and a unilateral vestibular and auditory function loss in one. None had angiographic evidence of arteriosclerotic disease of intracranial or extracranial cerebral arteries. An embolic explanation was favored by the focal nature of the neurological events, the involvement of both hemispheres at different times in three of the 12 patients, and the demonstration of occluded intracranial arteries in four patients despite normal extracranial arteries. These authors believe that "the process of thrombosis is involved with resultant embolism from the heart" but they lack pathological confirmation. They refer to Pomerance's (278) finding of tearing in the endocardium overlying the myxomatous valve and of adherent fibrin and red cells. According to this author (278) the endocardium overlying the redundant leaflets "which is subjected to abrupt changes in tension and resulting loss of endothelial continuity and rupture of subendothelial connective tissue fibers, would invite the deposition of fibrin seen in these cases." Heimbecker is quoted (21) as having observed at surgery a small thrombus lying on a myxomatous regurgitant valve near its attachment. In a subsequent article (203), the same group reported on 14 patients with TIA and MVP including the 12 cases previously published (21). Although they had not had any pathological confirmation in this group of patients, they published the pathological specimen of a middle aged woman who died suddenly while being investigated on a psychiatric ward and who had had atrial fibrillation and a murmur of mitral insufficiency: "A small adherent thrombus was found at necropsy at the base of a swollen, prolapsed posterior leaflet." They described a cul-de-sac between the left atrial wall and the prolapsed mitral leaflet providing the stasis necessary for thrombus formation particularly in the presence of atrial fibrillation. Others (380) also noted fibrinous deposits in the acute angle between the prolapsed posterior leaflet and the left atrial wall. In one of our patients, a 39-year-old woman who died suddenly (see Fig. 3.1) an ulceration was encountered in the same site without vegetations and without thrombus formation. We postulate that the ulceration may be due to overshooting of the prolapsed posterior leaflet with trauma to the left atrial wall. This ulceration could presumably be the site of thrombus formation. Three of the 12 patients reported by Barnett et al. (21) had paroxysmal atrial fibrillation, which may be responsible for left atrial thrombosis and cerebral embolus.

Barlow and Bosman (17) reported a transient left arm weakness in a 23-year-old woman with a recurrence 30 years later; midsystolic click and late systolic murmur were noted and MVP was evident on angiography. Leachman et al. (212) also reported in one patient a transient episode suggestive of hemiparesis that lasted 1 hr. I observed a transient hemiparesis in two young men with angiographically proven MVP, moderately severe mitral regurgitation, and no rhythm disturbance.

The relationship of idiopathic MVP and TIA poses a most intriguing problem and deserves further correlation and investigation by cardiologists and neurologists. An adequate auscultation and an echocardiogram should be recommended in all patients suffering from TIAs, not only to rule out mitral stenosis, and atrial myxoma, but also to determine if MVP is present.

PSYCHIATRIC MANIFESTATIONS

Symptoms of seemingly neuropsychiatric origin have been described in this syndrome (19,154,175). Hancock and Cohn (154) reported these symptoms in 15 of their 40 patients, including psychosis in four, hyperventilation syndrome in four, and psychoneurosis in seven. Fifteen patients out of 100 in our series (175) exhibited psychiatric manifestations, including psychoneurosis in seven, personality disorders in three, and psychosis in one. Munchausen's syndrome was noted in a patient with MVP (93). Shappell et al. (333) administered the Minnesota Multiphasic Personality Test (MMPI) to 14 patients known to have MVP and found abnormal scores in the six symptomatic ones: five had abnormal scores for hysteria and hypochondriasis, four abnormal scores for depression, psychopathic deviation and schizophrenia, and three abnormal scores for psychasthenia. The presence of normal MMPI in four symptomatic patients with aortic stenosis suggests that severe symptoms per se do not account for the abnormalities found in patients with the MVP syndrome. Psychoneurotic manifestations often precede clinical recognition of MVP and cannot, therefore, be considered as reactive or iatrogenic.

I concur with Wooley (394) that many of the patients previously described as suffering from Da Costa's syndrome, soldier's heart, the effort syndrome, and neurocirculatory asthenia would now be classified under the heading of MVP syndrome. Most of these patients complained of chest pain, effort dyspnea, fatigue, palpitations, dizziness, and exhibited heart deformities and asthenic body habitus. Barlow and Pocock (19) were impressed by the number of patients with MVP who appeared extremely anxious, some of whom fulfilled the criteria of Da Costa's syndrome or neurocirculatory asthenia.

Further investigation is needed to elucidate the significance of the psychiatric manifestations in this syndrome, their cause, and their true prevalence as compared to the general population. This should include auscultatory and echocardiographic screening of patients in mental institutions. These manifestations raise the possibility that the MVP syndrome is systemic rather than an isolated cardiac disease.

Chapter 6

Auscultatory and Phonocardiographic Findings

There are seven major auscultatory manifestations of idiopathic MVP syndrome (18,19,22,25,37,71,82,84,106,108,110,128,129,146,151,154,163, 169,175,178,195,209,231,249,260,264,276,283,287,300,303,310,319,320, 349,357,363,367,380,383,397) (Tables 6.1 and 6.2).

ISOLATED MID–LATE SYSTOLIC OR NONEJECTION CLICK

A snapping, crisp, high pitched mid–late systolic extra sound, is the auscultatory hallmark of this syndrome (Fig. 6.1). In some patients, it has a scratchy quality and in others it sounds like a systolic opening snap or may mimic the sound of a valvular prosthesis. In a few patients, it has the same pitch as normal heart sounds and can be distinguished from them only by its timing. Because of its high frequency, the click is best heard with the diaphragm of the stethoscope. As pointed out by Criley and Kissel (84), the casual auscultator may easily miss the click because "it may be assumed to be caused by a crackling of the stethoscope on the skin or bedclothes." Al-

TABLE 6.1. *Auscultatory manifestations in idiopathic MVP*

1. Isolated mid–late systolic click
2. Midsystolic click followed by a late systolic murmur
3. Early systolic click
4. Isolated late systolic murmur
5. Pansystolic murmur
6. Precordial honk or whoop
7. "Silent" MVP

TABLE 6.2. *Auscultatory and phonocardiographic findings in 350 patients followed by the author and his associates*

Isolated mid to late systolic click	186	(53.1%)
Early click	4	(1.1%)
Midsystolic click and late systolic murmur	60	(17.2%)
Late systolic murmur	7	(2.0%)
Precordial honk	4	(1. %)
Pansystolic murmur	30	(8.6%)
"Silent" MVP	59	(16.9%)
Total	350	(100%)

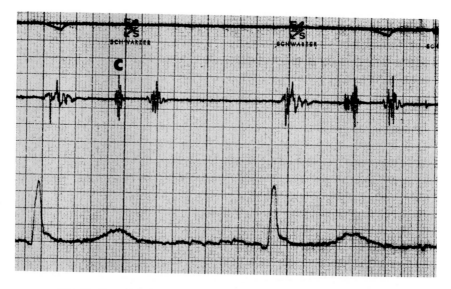

FIG. 6.1. *Case 45.* Isolated mid to late systolic click (c) in a 60-year-old woman.

though it is usually midsystolic, the click may occur late in systole to simulate a second sound-opening snap sequence (349) (Fig. 6.16). A carotid pulse, an apex cardiogram or various maneuvers (e.g., standing, amyl nitrite), might be needed to establish the diagnosis of late systolic click in these cases.

Multiple systolic clicks are often heard (in 24 of our first 100 patients) (175) (Fig. 6.2). To paraphrase Hancock and Cohn (154), when a well

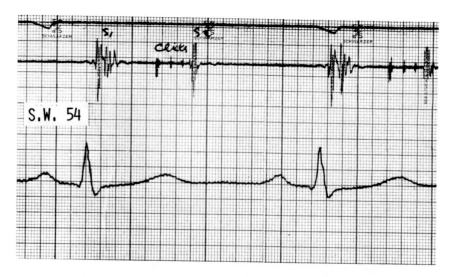

FIG. 6.2. *Case 87.* Multiple systolic clicks in a 54-year-old Chinese woman.

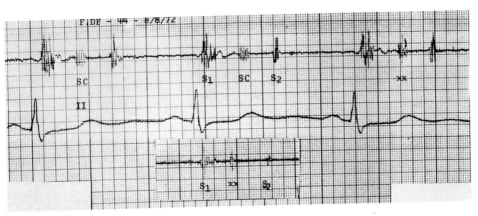

FIG. 6.3. *Case 100.* Proximity of two midsystolic clicks in a 44-year-old woman yielding a scratchy murmur that mimics the systolic component of a pericardial friction rub. SC, Summation click; x, Click. (From ref. 175. By permission)

trained house officer reports a "weird sounding heart," the likelihood is high that multiple clicks or precordial honks are present. As mentioned above, the auscultatory findings may be mistaken for the systolic component of a pericardial friction rub. The proximity of multiple clicks may yield a scratchy murmur, the way a diastolic rumble may result from the proximity of a third and fourth heart sound (175) (Fig. 6.3).

The click is best heard at the apex or inside the apex. In one recently reported case, the click was heard only over the left side of the neck in a 25-year-old woman with an echocardiogram diagnostic of MVP (106).

Clicks are often evanescent, vary from beat to beat and are independent of the respiratory cycle with regard to presence, timing, multiplicity, and association with murmur or honk (18,108,175,264). A click may not be present after various postural and pharmacological interventions have been tried on one examination, only to be prominent on another occasion (84). This characteristic of the click was well known to Cuffer and Barbillon (88), who pointed out that the click would come and go without apparent cause over periods of hours or days at a time.

Isolated click was noted in 186 of our 350 patients, in 21 of Barlow et al. 90 patients (18) and in 28 of Malcolm's 85 patients (231).

MIDSYSTOLIC CLICK FOLLOWED BY LATE SYSTOLIC MURMUR

This is a frequent combination that was noted in 60 of our 350 patients (Fig. 6.4). Barlow et al. (18) described these murmurs as crescendo–descrescendo, with maximal intensity occurring near the middle of the murmur in most patients, or very early or very late in a small number. The

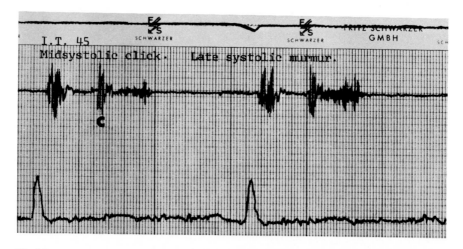

FIG. 6.4. Case 8. Apex phonocardiogram. Midsystolic click (c) followed by a late systolic murmur in a 48-year-old woman. See Fig. 8.6 for effect of amyl nitrite inhalation on EKG.

murmur always extends to the aortic component of the second sound and in some patients it extends beyond this sound. Other workers have described the murmur configuration as crescendo to the second sound (264). It classically begins with a click but it may precede the click and extend through it to the second sound. In some patients with a midsystolic click, an early to midsystolic murmur is heard and should be considered as an innocent murmur in these slender and young subjects (264).

The late systolic murmur is loudest at the apex and may be localized or transmitted to the axilla and the base (84). It is usually grade II–III/VI and increases in intensity in the left decubitus position (18). In some patients with isolated click in the supine position, a murmur can be elicited by changing posture to the left decubitus position, to sitting and leaning forward or standing (108,128).

EARLY SYSTOLIC CLICK

Early systolic click is an uncommon manifestation of this syndrome (163, 260). I encountered an isolated early systolic click in only four of my patients with MVP proven by echocardiography or angiography (Fig. 6.5). An early click is frequently noted, however, when multiple clicks are recorded (175).

Unlike the aortic ejection click that occurs before or at the onset of the upstroke of the carotid pulse tracing, the early click of MVP is usually recorded during the ascending limb of this tracing (260). However, some workers recorded early clicks of MVP before the carotid upstroke (163). In such a situation, the click of MVP can be distingiushed by its timing response to various maneuvers (amyl nitrite, standing, hand grip, etc.) and its variable relationship to the first heart sound and the carotid upstroke,

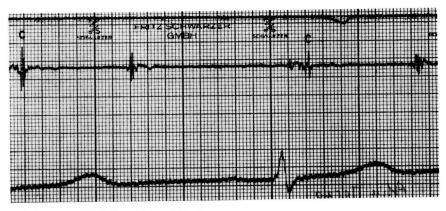

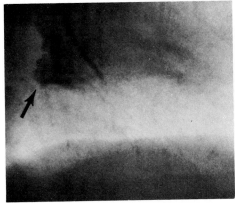

FIG. 6.5. *Case 325.* Early systolic click (c) in a 60-year-old patient with intractable chest pain and a normal coronary arteriogram. The diagnosis of MVP was confirmed by left cineventriculogram (RAO view), which showed prolapse of the posteromedial scallop of the posterior leaflet (arrow). See Fig. 8.14 for thallium scintigram.

indicating that the click is related to phenomena independent of aortic ejection. The early click of MVP may increase in intensity with inspiration, unlike the aortic ejection sound, which does not vary in intensity during the respiratory cycle and the pulmonic ejection sound, which increases in intensity on expiration (163).

Nasrallah et al. (260) correlated the early systolic click of MVP with the apex cardiogram and found it to occur after the apical ejection (E point) which coincides with the aortic ejection sound and at the onset of a second bulge that follows a systolic retraction.

Detection of an early click would warrant the diagnosis of idiopathic MVP only if corroborated by echocardiography (233) and/or left ventriculography (Figs. 6.5 and 9.3).

ISOLATED LATE SYSTOLIC MURMUR

Isolated late systolic murmur has been described as an auscultatory sign of MVP (18). It is, however, a nonspecific finding unless preceded by a click, and may occur in papillary muscle dysfunction, rheumatic mitral in-

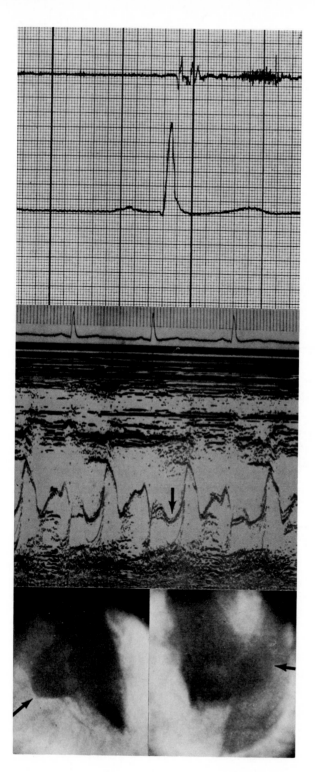

FIG. 6.6. Case 65. Isolated late systolic murmur in a 42-year-old man who complained of severe exertional chest pain. The diagnosis of MVP was confirmed by echocardiography, which showed mid-systolic dipping (arrow) and by left cineventriculography, which displayed massive prolapse of the posterior leaflet in both the RAO (A) and the LAO (B) views (arrows).

sufficiency, hypertrophic subaortic stenosis, and so forth (71,85,175,179). The late systolic murmur is due to late systolic mitral insufficiency resulting from "overshooting"(150) of prolapsed leaflets or scallops of posterior leaflet beyond the opposite number of the valve. The valve is competent at the beginning of systole but "leaks" at end systole. The dilated mitral annulus in MVP (46) may be another factor preventing apposition of the leaflets and allowing their prolapse into the left atrium, with overshooting and mitral regurgitation.

Response to various maneuvers may be helpful in implicating idiopathic MVP as a cause of the late systolic murmur. For instance, the late systolic murmur of rheumatic mitral regurgitation, unlike that of MVP, does not become holosystolic in the upright position. However, some of these maneuvers may elicit similar response in MVP and papillary muscle dysfunction on one hand (the murmur becomes pansystolic on standing and decreases in intensity on squatting), and in MVP and hypertrophic subaortic stenosis on the other (the murmur decreases in intensity on squatting). Echocardiographic and/or angiographic demonstration of MVP is required before attributing an isolated late systolic murmur to idiopathic MVP (Fig. 6.6). Unfortunately, several studies on the etiology and prognosis of idiopathic MVP have included a large number of patients with isolated late systolic murmurs, an inclusion that detracts from their conclusion (5,20,66).

PANSYSTOLIC MURMUR

Pansystolic murmur has been reported as the only auscultatory manifestation of MVP documented angiographically echocardiographically, or anatomically (Fig. 6.7). A late systolic murmur generally signifies mild mitral regurgitation (175). In our series, pansystolic murmur was noted in 30 out of 350 patients. The pansystolic murmur is often the manifestation of advanced idiopathic MVP, the so called "floppy mitral valve" (297) that is emerging as a major cause of pure mitral insufficiency (32,77,175,229,244, 306,319). I postulated that with advanced MVP, mitral regurgitation occurs throughout systole and the click can become masked by the loud pansystolic murmur or merge with the first heart sound (169,175). Floppy mitral valve is probably more common than rheumatic heart disease as an etiological factor in mitral insufficiency (304). Fifty out of 218 patients (23%) who underwent valve replacement for pure mitral insufficiency at Texas Heart Institute had floppy mitral valves (77). A higher prevalence of floppy mitral valve was reported by Salomon et al. (319): During a 9.5 year interval, 66 (49%) of 135 patients who had mitral valve replacement for pure mitral insufficiency were diagnosed as having myxomatous mitral valve on the basis of gross and histologic features of mitral valve tissue. Floppy mitral valve made up 9% (244) and 10% (108) respectively of all patients undergoing valve replacement in two institutions.

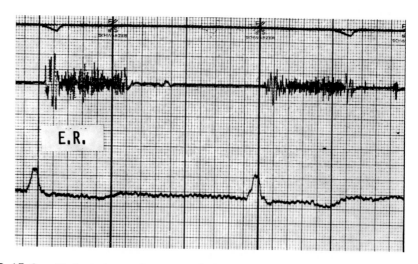

FIG. 6.7. Case 66. Apex phonocardiogram in a 56-year-old man with floppy mitral valve and severe mitral insufficiency, proven at surgery. A pansystolic murmur and a third heart sound were recorded. See Fig. 12.13 for left cineventriculogram. (From ref. 175. By permission)

Ruptured chordae tendineae was common in the three large series mentioned above [38% (77) 62% (319) 81% (244), respectively] but did not account for the mitral insufficiency and pansystolic murmur in all, since in one series (77) 55% had a history of heart murmur for a period up to 20 years and in another series (319) the preoperative interval during which a systolic murmur was known to be present averaged 14 years. In these series (77,244,319) that reported advanced MVP associated with mitral regurgitation, there was preponderance in males [53% (244) 56% (77) and 73% (319), respectively] that was not noted in other types of MVP.

In the presence of pure mitral insufficiency manifested by a pansystolic murmur, the diagnosis of MVP can only be made by echocardiography, left ventriculography, or on direct inspection of the mitral valve and microscopic analysis (150). However, the following clinical features would favor idiopathic mitral valve prolapse: late accentuation of the pansystolic murmur, absence of a loud first heart sound and of an opening snap, multiple premature ventricular contractions, T wave inversion in the inferior leads, and absence of mitral valve calcification.

In some patients with idiopathic MVP a midsystolic murmur is heard with or without a click. These murmurs are usually functional and innocent in these patients who have a high frequency of chest deformity. However, they may occupy all of systole in the upright position and in such a case they may represent mild mitral insufficiency. Another regurgitant murmur, the murmur of mild papillary muscle dysfunction, may be midsystolic in duration (155).

PRECORDIAL HONK OR WHOOP

A musical, loud, apical systolic murmur simulating the sound heard in whooping cough (246) or the honk made by a goose (287) has been described (Fig. 2.2). It is often isolated but can be superimposed on part of a systolic murmur (71). It is often transient and variable with position. Sitting, leaning forward, standing, or exercise might convert a late systolic murmur into a sonorous honk. The mitral origin of the honk was demonstrated by intracardiac phonocardiography (218) and the underlying MVP by means of left ventriculography (25,303) and echocardiography (125, 209,329,397). Minimal mitral regurgitation was usually evident (25). Cobbs (71) postulated resonation of a mitral leaflet to explain this curious sound: "A thin high velocity jet escaping from the edge of one prolapsed leaflet can probably sometimes strike tangentially the bulging surface of the other, acting like the bow of a violin."

This honk was intermittently heard in six of our patients. In all except two, MVP was demonstrated by the concomitant presence of a click, by echocardiography and/or angiography. Of the two remaining patients, one had primary cardiomyopathy with mitral insufficiency, and the other had coronary artery disease and ventricular aneurysm. The honk that can therefore be a manifestation of mitral insufficiency unrelated to idiopathic MVP (303) was also reported in a case of incompetence of a heterograft mitral valve associated with doming and prolapse of the leaflets (195). Moreover, in tricuspid insufficiency with or without demonstrable tricuspid prolapse, a honk has been heard (188,367).

Several patients with MVP stated that their own murmur had been audible to them on occasions (154). It can be assumed that on these occasions, a precordial honk was probably present (303). Several reports of "whistle" or honks heard across the room have appeared in the literature (209,265, 329,397). These include the case of a 12-year-old girl reported by Osler (265) who described a "remarkable whistling sound" that "was distinctly audible at a distance of three feet two inches by measurement and could be heard at any point of the chest and on top of the head." In the other three cases the loud variable honk was associated with a nonejection click and the echocardiogram was diagnostic of MVP in each instance.

In most patients with a honk, the abnormal sound has been heard since childhood.

"SILENT" MITRAL VALVE PROLAPSE

Acoustically "silent" MVP, a most intriguing form of this syndrome, deserves to be considered in the differential diagnosis of chest pain, arrhythmias, and ST-T abnormalities. In the absence of a click and/or murmur, MVP can be diagnosed by means of echocardiography and/or angiocardiography and

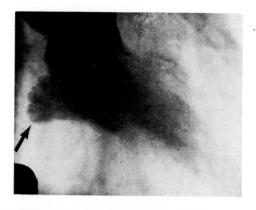

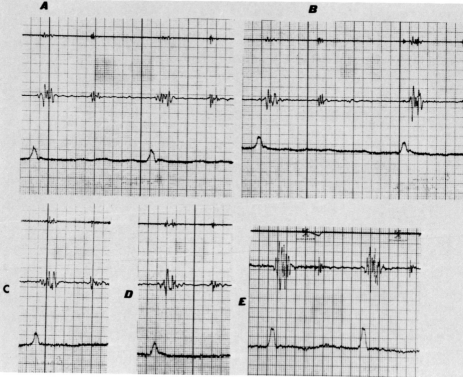

FIG. 6.8. *Case 144.* "Silent" MVP in a 40-year-old man who complained of severe chest pain. Coronary arteriogram showed no abnormalities. Phonocardiogram in the supine (A), left decubitus (B), sitting (C) and standing (D) positions, and after amyl nitrite inhalation (E) revealed neither click nor murmur. Left cineventriculogram in the RAO position: Prolapse of the posteromedial scallop of the posterior leaflet (arrow). Note hooded appearance. Echocardiogram showed a midsystolic buckling.

TABLE 6.3. *"Silent" MVP symptoms in 32 patients*

Chest pain	27
Dyspnea	15
Palpitations	13
Fatigue	10
Lightheadedness	8
Psychiatric symptoms	8
Syncope	3
Asymptomatic	2

is, therefore, termed "silent"(Figs. 6.8–6.13). Before designating MVP as "silent," auscultation in four positions (e.g., supine, left decubitus, sitting and standing) is required (Fig. 6.8). Various maneuvers, including squatting and amyl nitrite inhalation, should be utilized to elicit a click (233). In view of the evanescent nature of the nonejection click in some patients, auscultation should be carried out on various occasions, preferably by two observers before labeling a case as "silent." A phonocardiogram showing no click adds confirmatory evidence.

In 1969 I encountered my first case of angiographically proven MVP in whom neither click nor murmur were heard. I reported this case in 1971 and coined the term "silent ballooning" (169). Our group (178) subsequently reported on 32 cases of "silent MVP" demonstrated by angiography in ten cases, echocardiography in seven, and by both angiocardiography and echocardiography in 15 cases. This represented 16% of our total series of MVP which, at the time, stood at 207 cases. Nineteen patients were female and 13 were male. The mean age was 44. No patient had Marfan's syndrome. Most of these patients had been referred for evaluation of chest pain, which was present in 27 of them. Symptoms and EKG abnormalities in this group were similar to those encountered in typical cases of MVP associated with abnormal auscultatory findings (Tables 6.3 and 6.4). Selective coronary arteriography, which was performed in 22 patients, showed no abnormalities. Left ventriculography displayed prolapse of the posterior leaflet in 13 patients and of both leaflets in 12. We felt that "the silent form is not an uncommon presentation of the MVP syndrome, and that it should be sought in patients suffering from chest pain, particularly in the presence of a normal coronary arteriogram" (178).

TABLE 6.4. *"Silent" MVP electrocardiogram in 32 patients*

ST-T Changes in inferior leads	13
ST-T Changes in left precordial leads	5
ST-T Changes in right precordial leads	2
Ventricular irritability	5
Atrial fibrillation	3
Normal ECG	4

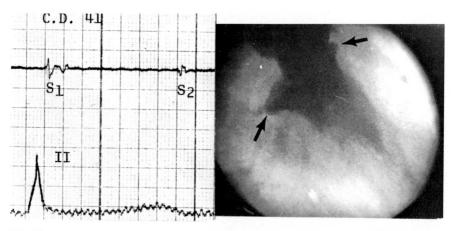

FIG. 6.9. *Case 69. Phono and LV cine in a 41-year-old man. Silent prolapse of both leaflets. Apex phono: no click. Cine LV: Prolapse of anterior leaflet (anterior hump sign as indicated by upper arrow) and posterior leaflet (posterior hump sign as indicated by lower arrow.) No MR. (From ref. 175. By permission)*

Other workers using echocardiographic criteria confirmed the frequent occurrence of silent MVP (45,99,100,231,233,282,283). However, Barlow and Pocock (19) disputed this concept, stating that in symptomatic or asymptomatic patients without abnormal auscultatory signs they have suspected MVP on the basis of abnormal EKG and "at a later examination such patients have frequently had a click or a late systolic murmur." They went on to say, "A few possibly have "silent prolapse" but in our opinion the auscultatory features would sooner or later be detected by careful and repeated auscultation."

To illustrate our findings in "silent MVP" two cases are briefly reported and electrocardiographic, angiographic, and echocardiographic data in other patients with this form are shown in Figs. 6.8,6.9,6.10, and 6.13.)

Case Reports
Case 1

A 21-year-old black female was referred with the chief complaint of mild nonexertional chest pain, dyspnea, fatigue, and premature ventricular beats on EKG. No clicks or murmurs were heard in various positions and following various maneuvers, including squatting and Valsalva maneuver. Cine left ventriculography in the RAO position was suggestive of MVP but the LAO view was diagnostic. The echocardiogram was indicative of MVP. (Fig. 6.11)

Case 2

A 32-year-old white female gave a history of multiple hospital admissions and monitoring in the coronary care unit for severe nonexertional chest pain and an abnormal EKG showing evanescent ST-T changes. No clicks or murmurs were heard in various positions. Cine left ventriculogram in the RAO view was suggestive of prolapse but the LAO view was diagnostic. Coronary arteriogram showed no abnormalities. The echocardiogram was not technically satisfactory. The patient responded well to reassurance and propranolol and has not required hospitalization in four years. (Fig. 6.12)

On the basis of published reports and of my own observations, I am convinced that the "silent" form of idiopathic MVP is not uncommon. Despite postural and pharmacological interventions, auscultation and phonocardiography reveals no abnormalities in 10 to 15% of patients with echocar-

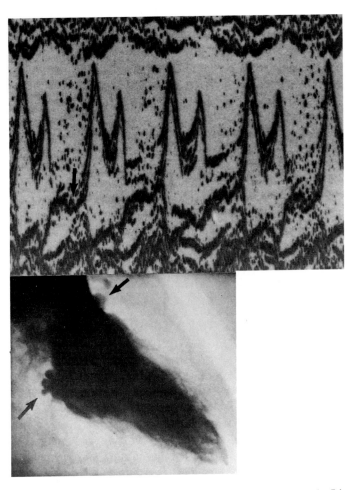

FIG. 6.10. *Case 187.* "Silent" MVP in a 46-year-old woman with severe chest pain. Echocardiogram shows midsystolic buckling (arrow). Left cineventriculogram in the RAO position shows prolapse of a multi-scalloped posterior leaflet. Lower arrow points to posteromedial scallop and upper arrow to either the anterior leaflet or the anterolateral scallop of the posterior leaflet.

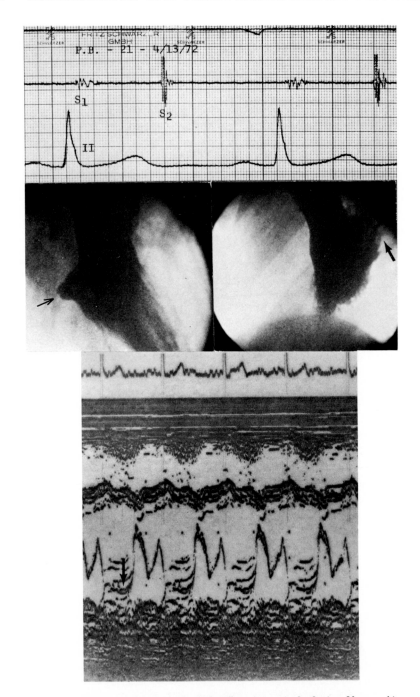

FIG. 6.11. *Case 50.* Silent prolapse of posteromedial scallop of posterior leaflet in a 21-year-old woman. Apex phonocardiogram shows no click. LV cine in RAO position (A) shows minimal prolapse of the postero-medial scallop of the posterior leaflet (arrow). This angiographic appearance may represent a normal variant. However, the LAO view (B) shows a marked protrusion diagnostic of MVP (arrow). The echo-cardiogram demonstrates a midsystolic buckling diagnostic of MVP. (From refs. 171 and 181. By permission)

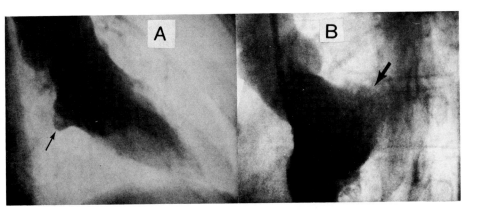

FIG. 6.12. *Case 190.* Left cineventriculogram in a 32-year-old woman with silent MVP (see text). A. RAO view shows minimal prolapse of the posteromedial (lower arrow) scallop of the posterior leaflet. B. LAO view. The prolapse of the posterior leaflet is more conspicuous in this view (arrow). Note anterior displacement of the apex which is aligned with the left atrium (See Fig. 8.8 for EKG).

diographic and/or angiographic prolapse. The mechanism of absence of click and/or murmur has not been elucidated. To avoid labeling patients as having heart disease, albeit with a generally benign course, we should adhere to the following rigid criteria in making the diagnosis of silent MVP:

1. Echocardiographic diagnosis should be made only if midsystolic buckling is noted or if pansystolic sagging of 3 mm and preferably 5 mm is evident. Only the "perpendicular" transducer position should be used when analyzing the echocardiogram for the presence of MVP.

2. The angiographic findings that will be discussed later should be obvious and should not be limited to minimal "lipping." Normal variants including accumulation of dye in the fornix of the mitral valve should not be mistakenly diagnosed as indicative of MVP. In some patients the left anterior oblique position can be more diagnostic than the right anterior oblique position and the two positions should be used often (Figs. 6.11 and 6.12). The cinematographic motion of the valve should be observed because of the characteristic appearance when prolapse is present.

I have already discussed the nonspecificity of the angiographic features of idiopathic MVP and their frequent occurrence in coronary artery disease as a manifestation of papillary muscle dysfunction. It is possible that in some patients an angiographic picture reminiscent of idiopathic MVP could be caused by a yet undefined disorder of the papillary muscle including focal myocardial involvement, small coronary artery disease, old infarction in the presence of normal coronary arteries, and so forth. I would, therefore, urge that in the absence of a click the angiographic diagnosis should be confirmed by echocardiography. However, it is not always possible to obtain technically adequate echocardiogram, and even if an adequate echocardiogram is ob-

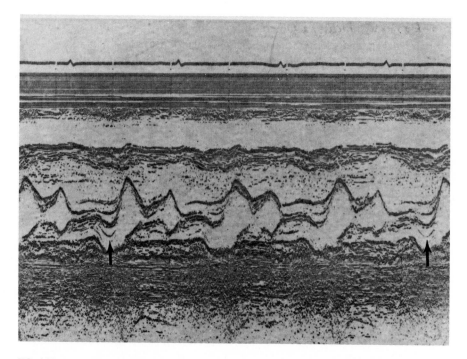

FIG. 6.13. *Case 330*. Echocardiogram in a young woman with "silent" MVP. The tracing which shows a midsystolic buckling is diagnostic of MVP. Note that the most posterior echo is the less intense and can be missed if the gain is too low (arrows).

tained, it could be false negative in idiopathic MVP. In view of these considerations, the diagnosis of idiopathic MVP can be made in an occasional patient on the basis of angiographic features alone if these features are clear-cut. This diagnosis should be correlated with the clinical picture including symptoms and EKG abnormalities.

MECHANISM OF PRODUCTION OF THE CLICK AND MURMUR

Criley et al. (85), using nonsimultaneous cineangiographic–phonocardiographic correlation showed that the click coincides with the time of maximal mitral valve prolapse. Winkle et al. (383) confirmed these observations by echo–phonocardiographic studies that revealed that the peak intensity of the click usually coincides with the point of maximal prolapse. The click was attributed by Reid (298) to sudden tightening of the chordae in midsystole, the "chordal snap." Lewis (221) ascribed it to "sudden tensing of the everted valve leaflet," "snapping of a sail" phenomenon. This theory was confirmed by Dock (110), who reproduced a click by lateral tensing of the isolated anterior mitral cusp that had been removed from the heart. However, Craige (82), subscribing to a unitarian theory on the genesis of the heart sounds that has recently gained considerable support in the literature has attributed the click to "sudden deceleration of a mass of blood with resultant vibrations involving the heart chambers, valves and contents."

Multiple clicks may be due to asynchronous prolapse of either the leaflets or the scallops of the posterior leaflet (380).

CLICKS IN OTHER MITRAL DISORDERS AND IN DISEASES NOT INVOLVING THE MITRAL VALVE APPARATUS

An early systolic click was reported in small ventricular defects associated with aneurysmal formation (273,274). Pickering and Keith (273) postulated that the sound was "produced in much the same way as the sound of a sail when it catches the wind." However, none of these patients underwent left ventriculography in the RAO position to rule out associated MVP. I have not observed a click in six patients who had aneurysm of the ventricular septum. Clicks and whoops have been described in left sided pneumothorax, but they are usually multiple, occur in both systole and diastole (309), and vary with both inspiration and position. Other features of pneumothorax are apparent.

A systolic tumor sound was described in calcified atrial myxoma (235), and is probably the systolic equivalent of the so called "tumor plop." A midsystolic click was also described in a case of paradoxic embolism extending from the patent foramen ovale into the left atrium and across the mitral valve into the left ventricle (323). The mitral valve leaflets were normal and "movement of thrombus from ventricle toward atrium during systole may have played a role in the genesis of the midsystolic click."

A pseudo-ejection sound associated with systolic anterior motion of the anterior mitral leaflet on the echocardiogram was described in hypertrophic subaortic stenosis (356). This sound was later in systole than the aortic ejection sound, beginning 40 to 100 msec after the upstroke of the indirect carotid pulse and occurring close to the initial peak of the carotid pulse.

Post mitral valvotomy nonejection clicks have been described (18) but are quite uncommon. I have not heard them in our post valvotomy patients. It is possible that the stenosis in patients who developed clicks after valvotomy may have been superimposed on a myxomatous redundant valve; the commissurotomy by freeing the leaflets may then allow these abnormal leaflets to generate a click.

The probable coincidental association of MVP and mitral stenosis was reported in four patients, two of whom underwent mitral valve surgery (352). However, no comment was made on the postoperative auscultatory findings.

Clicks and/or late systolic murmur due to tricuspid valve prolapse have been described (143,393). Intracardiac phonocardiography (393) in a young woman with documented MVP and a left heart nonejection click and late systolic murmur showed a right heart click and late systolic murmur that were augmented by inspiration and recorded from the right atrium in proximity to the tricuspid valve. Right ventricular cineangiography demonstrated prolapse of the tricuspid valve with minimal tricuspid regurgitation. However, the published intracardiac sound study showed only a late systolic murmur. In another report on tricuspid valve prolapse (143), the clinical clue to tricuspid valve prolapse associated with MVP was the transient appearance at the left lower sternal border of a late systolic murmur after deep inspiration. During normal breathing only an apical murmur and midsystolic click could be heard.

RESPONSE OF THE CLICK AND MURMUR TO VARIOUS MANEUVERS

As previously pointed out, the click is not always evident in the supine position. Auscultation should be carried out in at least four positions (e.g., supine, left decubitus, sitting, and standing), in order to detect it (128) (Figs. 6.14 and 6.15). In some patients with isolated clicks, a late systolic murmur can be induced by various maneuvers.

The timing of the click is affected by changes in left ventricular volume and contractility (9,18,84,127,129,175,264,322,332) (Table 6.5, Fig. 6.16). Mathey et al. (242) studied the determinants of onset of MVP by analyzing echocardiograms and simultaneously recorded phonocardiograms. They demonstrated that the click occurs at a critical left ventricular volume and that the left ventricular chamber size at which the prolapse occurred was "virtually constant for an individual patient." With a smaller left ventricular end-diastolic volume, the leaflets tend to be closer to a position of prolapse and the latter is attained shortly after the onset of contraction: the converse is true with a larger end-diastolic volume. A change in left ventricular contractility is another factor responsible for the variability of timing of the click: an increase in the velocity of the fiber shortening in the preprolapse period results in earlier timing and a decrease has the opposite effect. The murmur, when present, follows the click, becoming late when the click moves toward the second heart sound and becoming almost pansystolic when the click moves toward and even merges with the first heart sound (Table 6.6). Maneuvers such as inspiration, standing, tilt, Valsalva maneuver, amyl nitrite inhalation, pacing (363), or isoproterenol, which induce a decrease in left ventricular volume, result in early occurrence of the click and the murmur. (Figs. 6.16, 6.17, 6.18, and 6.20). Opposite maneuvers such as squatting, propranolol, or phenylephrine delay their occurrence. Amyl nitrite (Fig. 6.17) induces earlier onset of the click and murmur by acting through two mechanisms: decrease in left ventricular volume and increase in left ventricular contractility. I showed that isometric hand grip exercise causes the click and the murmur to move toward the second sound (175) and others

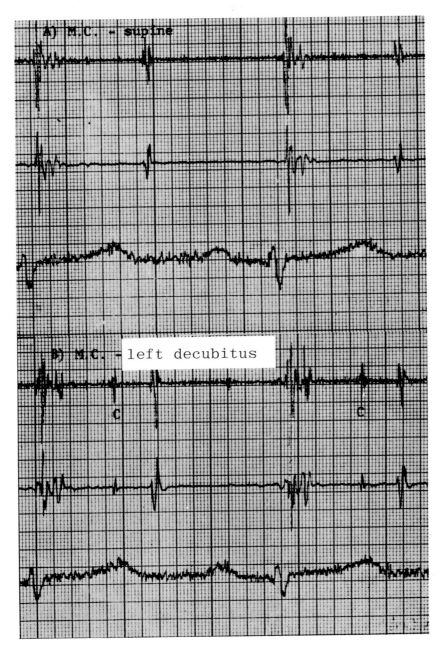

FIG. 6.14. Case 174. Apex phonocardiogram in the supine and in the left decubitus positions in a 56-year-old woman. A mid–late systolic click (c) was noted only in the left decubitus position. Left cineventriculogram (Fig. 12.26) showed MVP.

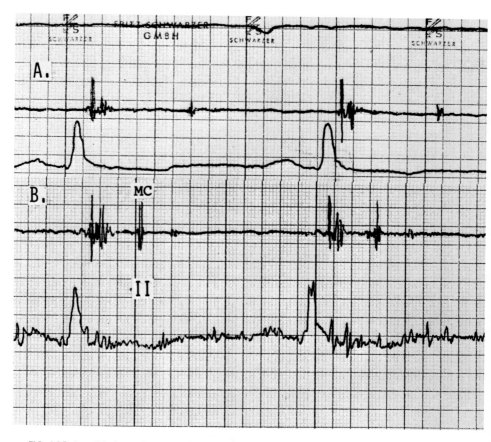

FIG. 6.15. *Case 26. Apex phonocardiogram in a 49-year-old man. A. In the supine position no click is recorded. B. In the standing position a midsystolic click is recorded. See Fig. 8.2. (From ref. 169. By permission)*

(332) had noted a similar effect (Figs. 6.18 and 6.19). However, O'Rourke and Crawford (264) postulated that the increase in heart rate and in cardiac contractility associated with hand grip would have the opposite effect but they stated that more severe degree of hand grip may result "in more variable changes in the systolic click-murmur complex."

In premature ventricular contractions, the ventricular diastolic diameter is reduced and the click and murmur move toward the first heart sound. The same phenomenon was also reported with atrial premature beats (300). The paradoxical early occurrence of the click and murmur in post extra systolic beats (242) and after termination of rapid atrial pacing (363) despite the increase in left ventricular volume can be explained by the increase in the velocity of circumferential fiber shortening in the preprolapse period.

In some patients with isolated pansystolic murmurs as a manifestation of

TABLE 6.5. *Effects of various maneuvers on timing of click and murmur*

	S_1	S_2
Inspiration	←—	
Standing	←—	
Tilt	←—	
Valsalva	←—	
Amyl nitrite	←—	
PVC	←—	
Pacing	←—	
Post extrasystolic beat	←—	
Squatting	—→	
Hand grip	—→	
Pressor agents	—→	
Propranolol	—→	
Passive leg raising	—→	

MVP and mitral regurgitation, the hand grip test, squatting, or vasoactive substances by delaying prolapse may unmask an early click merged with the first heart sound or "buried" within the murmur, and make the murmur late systolic in timing and preceded by a click (175).

The effects of various maneuvers on the timing of the click is helpful in the diagnosis of MVP, particularly when an early or a late systolic click is heard. Unlike ejection sounds, the early click of MVP can be "maneuvered" away from the first heart sound. The late systolic click can be so close to the second sound as to be superficially mistaken for a split S2; the sequence click–second sound can also be mistaken for second sound–opening snap. However, the various maneuvers, which reduce left ventricular size, displace the click toward midsystole, thus identifying its true nature (Fig. 6.17). The intensity of the click was shown to increase "in all instances of potentiation of contractility" (363).

The intensity of regurgitant murmur in this syndrome varies with the level of arterial pressures, increasing with maneuvers that raise this pressure (vasopressors) and becoming softer with those that decrease it (early phase of amyl nitrite inhalation). However, left ventricular volume both at end-diastole and end systole influences the timing and degree of prolapse. No MVP and hence no mitral insufficiency and no murmurs would occur if the ventricular volume at the end of systole does not reach the critical prolapse volume; on the other hand significant pansystolic mitral insufficiency would result from a small left ventricular diastolic volume with excessive systolic emptying. With a decreased left ventricular diastolic volume, the leaflets are closer to a position of prolapse as just mentioned. A reduced left ventricular end systolic volume causes "the chordae to become too long relative to the axis of the chamber" (66), and permits the leaflet "to billow into the left atrium before tensing of the chordae could check its advance" (170). This would favor more pronounced prolapse and mitral regurgitation.

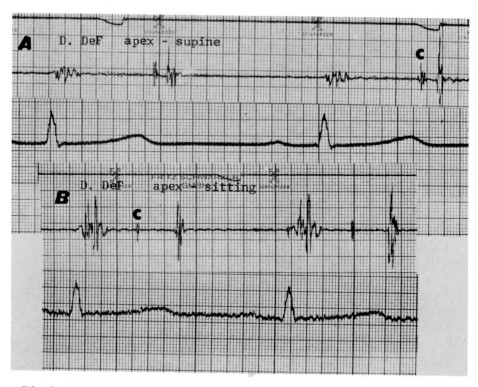

FIG. 6.16. *Case 86.* Apex phonocardiogram: Effect of sitting position on timing of click in a 39-year-old woman. A. Supine position. A late systolic click (c) was recorded. B. Sitting position. The click (c) has moved to midsystole.

The effects of various maneuvers on the intensity of the murmur in an individual patient depend on the interaction of two factors: arterial systolic pressure and degree and duration of prolapse as influenced by left ventricular volume. Squatting, for instance, despite the increase in blood pres-

TABLE 6.6. *Effects of various maneuvers on the murmur in idiopathic MVP*

INTERVENTIONS	MURMUR
Inspiration	Earlier onset, louder
Standing	Earlier onset, louder
Squatting	Later onset, softer or absent
Hand grip	Variable onset and intensity
Passive leg raising	Later onset, softer
Valsalva (strain phase)	Earlier onset—variable intensity
Valsalva (release)	Later onset—variable intensity
Amyl nitrite	Earlier onset—softer initially and louder subsequently
Methoxamine, phenylephrine	Later or no change, louder
Propranolol	Later, softer or absent

Modified from ref. 127.

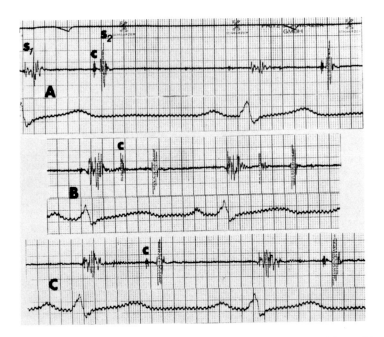

FIG. 6.17. *Case 72.* Effect of amyl nitrite (AN) inhalation on the timing of the click (c) in a 27-year-old man. A. Apex phono in the supine position: Early and late systolic clicks. B. After AN inhalation, the late systolic click moves earlier, and in (C) it returns to its previous position when the effect of AN had subsided. (From ref. 175. By permission)

sure that would be expected to increase the intensity of the murmur, is usually associated with a softening or abolition of the murmur because this maneuver increases venous return, slows the heart rate and hence increases left ventricular volume (Fig. 6.21). Fontana et al. (129) pointed out that the increase in left ventricular volume "would produce more tension on the mitral valve leaflets and chordae by increasing the distance between the ventricular wall and the papillary muscles and valve ring. Later and less leaflet prolapse would then result during systole." Amyl nitrite inhalation because of a drop in blood pressure produces a decrease in intensity of the murmur in MVP within 15 to 30 sec. However, because MVP is longer and more pronounced due to decreased left ventricular volume and excessive emptying, the murmur returns to louder than the control within 45 to 60 sec (9). Indeed, cineangiography after amyl nitrite inhalation has shown the mitral regurgitation to be earlier in onset and greater in magnitude (32). The intensity of the murmur increases in the upright position and at 45° despite the drop in blood pressure. This is due to decreased left ventricular end-diastolic and end-systolic volume, leading to greater prolapse (63). A greater degree of prolapse was also shown by cineangiography in the 45°, head up, tilt position (129).

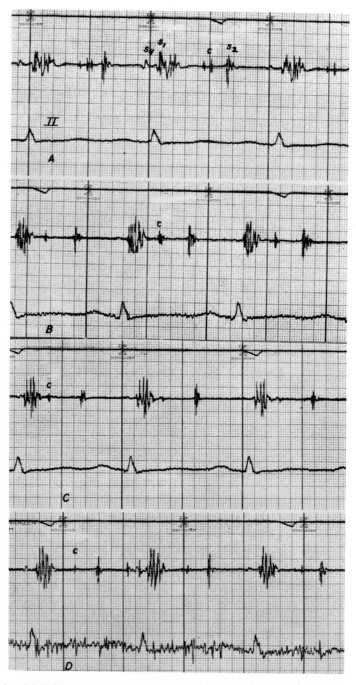

FIG. 6.18. Case 78. Multiple clicks in a 32-year-old woman. Effect of various positions and hand grip test on timing of click. A. Apex phono in the supine position: Multiple clicks (c) and S_4 (fourth heart sound.) B. Sitting position: The click moves towards the first heart sound. C. Standing position: The click moves closer to the first heart sound. D. Hand grip test in the standing position: A fourth heart sound is recorded and the click moves towards the second heart sound. (From ref. 175. By permission)

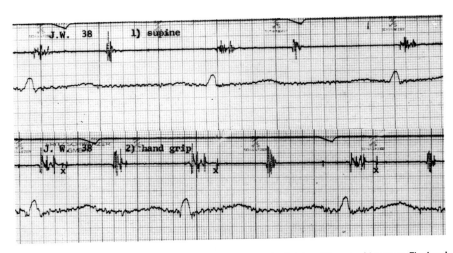

FIG. 6.19. Case 124. Effect on hand grip maneuver on an early click in a 38-year-old woman. The hand grip either unmasks a new click (x) or moves it away from the first heart sound.

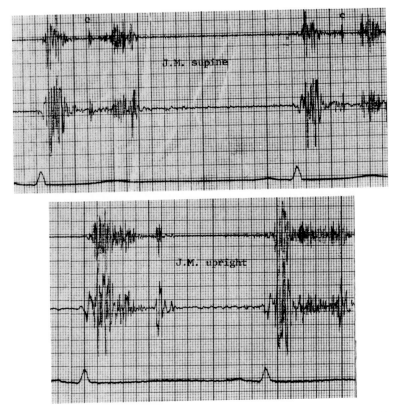

FIG. 6.20. Case 184. Effect of upright position on click and murmur in a 27-year-old woman. Standing: Midsystolic click (c) followed by a late systolic murmur. Upright: Murmur becomes pansystolic and masks click.

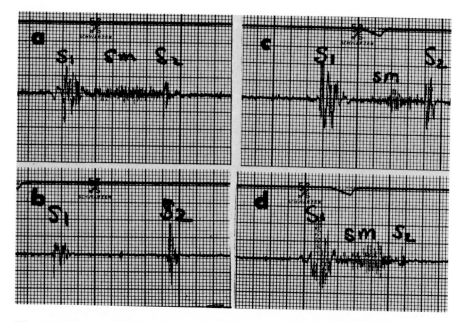

FIG. 6.21. Effect of standing (a) squatting (b), and amyl nitrite inhalation on the murmur in a young woman with late systolic murmur in the supine position (c) and an echocardiogram indicative of MVP. a. Standing: The murmur becomes pansystolic. b. squatting: The murmur is no longer evident. c. Supine: Late systolic murmur. d. Amyl nitrite inhalation in the supine position; the murmur becomes pansystolic and louder. S_1, First heart sound. S_2, Second heart sound. PM, Pansystolic murmur. LSM, Late systolic murmur.

Use of Maneuvers in Differential Diagnosis

The effect of various maneuvers on the timing and intensity of the murmur in idiopathic MVP is shown in Table 6.6. It should be stressed that there are frequent individual variations (127) due to the sum of opposing influences such as blood pressure and left ventricular volume. The volume related response of the murmur to various interventions is helpful in identifying MVP and in differentiating it from rheumatic mitral insufficiency but not from papillary muscle dysfunction and idiopathic hypertrophic subaortic stenosis (IHSS). The change in intensity resembles that which is observed in IHSS (i.e., decreased intensity on squatting and increased intensity in the upright position). Although the murmur in both MVP and IHSS increases in intensity after amyl nitrite inhalation, early softening of the murmur is observed only in MVP. The Valsalva maneuver is followed by a great increase in the intensity of the murmur in IHSS in contrast to the murmur of MVP, which becomes longer but not necessarily louder (264). The mitral insufficiency in papillary muscle dysfunction is often due to prolapse into the left atrium of normal nonmyxomatous mitral leaflets poorly anchored by the ischemic or infarcted papillary muscles. Therefore, both in idiopathic

MVP and in papillary muscle dysfunction the response of the murmur to maneuvers and interventions is volume and pressure related.

Amyl nitrite inhalation and squatting are the two procedures most helpful in differentiating the murmur of idiopathic MVP from that of rheumatic mitral regurgitation: the murmur in MVP increases with amyl nitrite following an initial decrease but it softens in rheumatic mitral regurgitation. On prompt squatting, the murmur increases in rheumatic mitral regurgitation but decreases in MVP.

The murmur of aortic stenosis increases after amyl nitrite inhalation, usually decreases in intensity during the straining phase of the Valsalva maneuver, and has a variable response to squatting (310). These maneuvers, therefore, do not help differentiate it from the murmur of MVP. The diagnosis should be based on duration of the murmur, its transmission, and other findings on physical examination.

In summary, the timing response of the murmur of MVP to various maneuvers is helpful in the differential diagnosis except in papillary muscle dysfunction. However, the variability of the intensity of the response of the murmur precludes the use of this response in the differential diagnosis, except in rheumatic mitral regurgitation.

EFFECT OF PREGNANCY ON THE MIDSYSTOLIC CLICK AND MURMUR

Haas (151) reported on the alterations of the auscultatory findings of the midsystolic click–late systolic murmur during gestation in three patients. In two, the systolic click and the late systolic murmur disappeared whereas in the third only the click persisted. The author attributed these changes to the increased blood volume and left ventricular end-diastolic volume during pregnancy and to the reduction in peripheral resistance. I would favor the volumetric explanation in the two patients who lost both click and murmur, postulating that the left ventricular end systolic volume in these patients may have exceeded the "critical" prolapse volume. In the patient who lost the murmur only, the drop in blood pressure and the increase in volume would explain this finding. Sasse (320) reported a move of the click and murmur to early systole in a pregnant patient despite the increase in echocardiographic left ventricular diastolic and systolic volume as compared to prepregnancy.

DIASTOLIC SOUNDS ASSOCIATED WITH MVP

An early diastolic sound associated with idiopathic MVP has been reported (37,69,73,154,254) in the absence of mitral stenosis and was noted in two of my patients. Cobbs and King (73) presented evidence suggesting that this extra sound was the pulmonary component of a widely split S2.

However, Cheng (69) was able to identify, on expiration, the pulmonary component of the second sound between the aortic component and the "diastolic click." Others have shown that the diastolic sound coincides approximately with the 0 point of the apex cardiogram (154) and with the E point of the mitral valve echogram (254). These features would identify the sound as an opening snap of a nonstenotic mitral valve. However, Bonner et al. (37), using simultaneous echo–phonocardiographic and phono–apex cardiographic recordings, demonstrated that the sound occurred "well before both the E point of the mitral valve echogram and the 0 point of the apex cardiogram." There was no evidence of mitral stenosis or atrial septal defect on the echocardiogram in their patients. They ascribed the extra sound to lateral tension of the leaflet as it accelerates from its prolapsed position toward the left ventricular cavity.

It is evident that considerable controversy surrounds the mechanism and origin of the diastolic sound in MVP. This sound should be differentiated from the opening snap of mitral stenosis and from the wide and fixed splitting of the second sound of atrial septal defect that is frequently associated with MVP. Cheng states, "Diastolic click in MVP should now be added to the list of different causes of a "third heard sound" which in order of its temporal proximity to the second sound are: physiological duplication of a second sound, opening snap of mitral stenosis, tumor plop of left atrial myxoma, diastolic knock of constrictive pericarditis and diastolic gallop" (69). To my knowledge this diastolic sound has not been described in the absence of a systolic click or in "silent MVP."

Chapter 7

Other Physical and Graphic Findings in MVP

The general physical appearance in idiopathic MVP may be entirely normal. However, certain features (e.g., asthenic body habitus, high arched palate, thoracic bony abnormalities such as straight back, pectus excavatum) are frequently noted in this syndrome and heighten suspicion of idiopathic MVP (38,85,318).

INCREASED JOINT LAXITY

Increased joint laxity was reported by Evans et àl. (119) in ten subjects with MVP. Joint mobility was determined by multiple X-ray views of passive displacement of the metacarpal–phalangeal joint of the left index finger. There was a statistically significant increase in posterior displacement in patients with MVP. This abnormality could not be confirmed by Perloff (272) who examined his patients specifically for lax ligaments. The true prevalence and significance of joint laxity in MVP awaits further studies.

PRECORDIAL PALPATION AND APEX CARDIOGRAM

In the absence of significant mitral regurgitation the heart is not enlarged on palpation and no apical heave is felt. Apex cardiogram frequently shows a sharp midsystolic retraction coinciding with the midsystolic click (19,104, 118,231,343,362) that is accentuated by standing and amyl nitrite inhalation (343). To explain this retraction, Pocock and Barlow (276) suggested that "abnormal tension on an ischemic papillary muscle could result in the base of the muscle being drawn inward." The double peaked apex cardiogram during systole resembles that seen in hypertrophic subaortic stenosis (104,362), myocardial infarction, angina pectoris, ventricular aneurysm (362), and atrial myxoma. On precordial palpation, it is occasionally noted in the left decubitus position (19,362).

CAROTID PULSE TRACING

Midsystolic retraction of the carotid pulse recording has been reported in MVP (27). This systolic retraction occurs during or after recording of the midsystolic click and tends to move earlier with assumption of the upright position and following inhalation of amyl nitrite. It has been attributed to abrupt midsystolic left ventricular decompression secondary to the MVP and may mimic the bifid carotid pulse tracing that is noted in hypertrophic sub-aortic stenosis.

Systolic retraction of the aortic valve echocardiogram was observed by Howard et al. (159) in MVP in the absence of obstruction of the left ventricular outflow tract. It was shown to coincide with the inscription of the click and with the systolic retraction on left ventricular apex cardiogram and on external carotid pulse tracing.

DERMATOGLYPHIC PATTERNS IN PATIENTS WITH MVP (FIG. 7.1)

Swartz et al. (354) studied the fingerprints in 100 patients with MVP and compared them with 100 control subjects matched for sex and race. The dermatoglyphic complex patterns are classified into three main groups: whorls, loops, and arches. Arches that are composed of a succession of gently curving ridges were found in 16.8% of all digital patterns in patients with MVP but in only 2.5% of the control group. Patients with MVP had a higher percentage of four or more arches. Moreover, arches on digits IV and V were found exclusively in patients with MVP. These authors felt that the finding of four or more arches on digits IV and V may be an important supportive evidence of MVP. They suspected antenatal factors in the pathogenesis of MVP and postulated that a genetic or environmental factor that interferes with the development of the mitral valve may also influence epidermal ridge patterns that bear a close temporal relationship in their embryological formation. Bon Tempo et al.

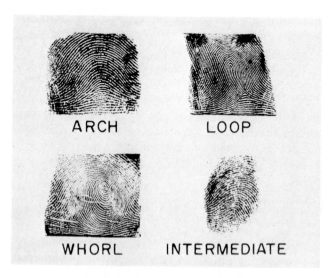

FIG. 7.1. Examples of fingerprint patterns.
(From ref. 354. Courtesy of M. H. Swartz et al. and by permission of *Am J Cardiology.*)

(38), who had encountered a high prevalence of thoracic bony abnormalities in MVP, suggested a similar embryologic explanation since the vertebral column and thoracic cage begin their chondrification and ossification at the time that the mitral valve undergoes differentiation. This intriguing association of MVP with dermatoglyphic patterns awaits confirmation by other workers.

Chapter 8

Electrocardiographic Features, Arrhythmias, and Conduction Defects

Electrocardiographic abnormalities, arrhythmias, and conduction defects are frequently encountered in idiopathic MVP and have been the subject of numerous investigations and publications. (1,19,33,42,49,52,53,60,71,76,84, 98,103,108,122,134,135,144,149,154,165,169,175,183,211,217,226,228, 230,231,234,258,264,275,276,283,301,321,322,326,355,358,359,366,380, 385,386,392,398,399). Sudden death, a rare occurrence in this syndrome, is generally felt to be arrhythmic in origin, and will be discussed in Chap. 14.

Humphries and McKusick (161) were the first to draw attention to the electrocardiographic abnormalities, coining the term "auscultatory-electrocardiographic syndrome," but they mistakenly felt that these changes were the "residue of pericarditis." Barlow and associates (18) described in detail the ST -T changes associated with this syndrome.

The typical electrocardiographic abnormalities consist of low, initially or totally inverted T waves in leads II, III, and AVF with or without minimal ST depression (175) (Figs. 8.1 to 8.3). These changes were noted in 42 of my first 100 patients, initial T wave inversion being the most common anomaly ˙(175). Twenty-four of these 42 patients had similar changes in the left precordial leads, and 10 in the right precordial leads (Fig. 8.4). T wave changes in the right precordial leads were associated with prolapse of both leaflets (7 out of 100 patients). In the 26 patients who had a normal coronary arteriogram, the EKG was abnormal in 16 with ST -T abnormalities in the inferior leads in all, with associated changes in the left precordial leads in eight and in the right precordial leads in five (175). Of 144 patients studied by Barlow and Pocock (19), 53 (37%) had an abnormal EKG, 32 of whom had the most widely recognized pattern of inverted or partially inverted T waves in the inferior leads. The same workers described the ST segment as being usually normal, slightly elevated, or only mildly depressed. They also encountered similar T wave abnormalities in the anterior leads. A similar occurrence of ST -T abnormalities was described by Lardani et al. (211), who detected these abnormalities in 37% of 145 patients with angiographically proven MVP. They found no relationship between the severity of the MVP and the EKG changes. Other workers (85,128,144,154,226,282,357) reported ST -T abnormalities predominantly in the inferior leads and also in the right precordial leads (149,226,260) in the absence of coronary artery disease. Unlike others

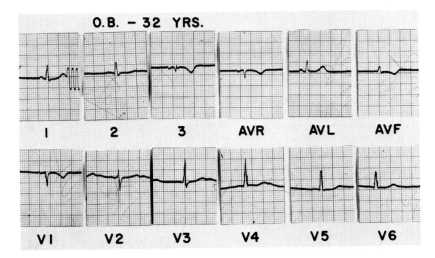

FIG. 8.1. *Case 12.* T wave inversion in the inferior leads in a 32-year-old woman with a midsystolic click and late systolic murmur. Note prominent U waves.

(276), we noted abnormal T waves in 13 patients who had "silent" prolapse and normal selective coronary arteriograms.

The true prevalence of ST -T abnormalities in subjects prospectively examined for the presence of MVP is much lower than that reported by cardiac referral centers: 15% in Procacci et al.'s survey (286) and 18% in Markiewicz

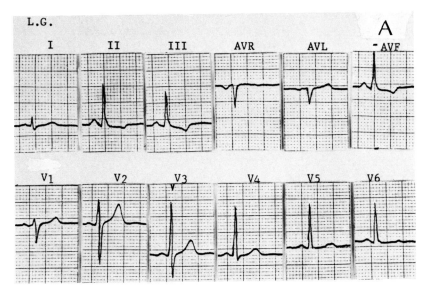

FIG. 8.2. *Case 26.* MVP and EKG abnormalities in a 49-year-old man who complained of atypical chest pain. MSC was heard only in the standing position. (Fig. 6.15) The EKG (A) shows ST depression and T inversion in II, III, and AVF, and flat T waves in V₆. The T waves are tall in the midprecordial leads. MSC, Mid-systolic click.

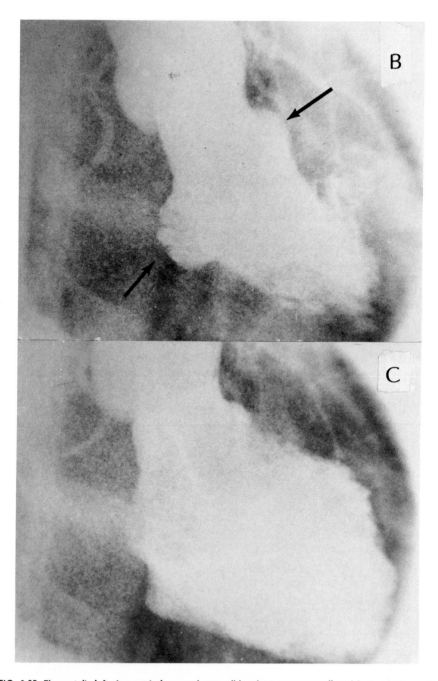

FIG. 8.2B. The systolic left cineventriculogram shows a "doughnut appearance" and both anterior and rounded posterior "hump sign" (*arrows*). C. Diastole (See Fig. 6.15). (From refs. 169 and 175. By permission)

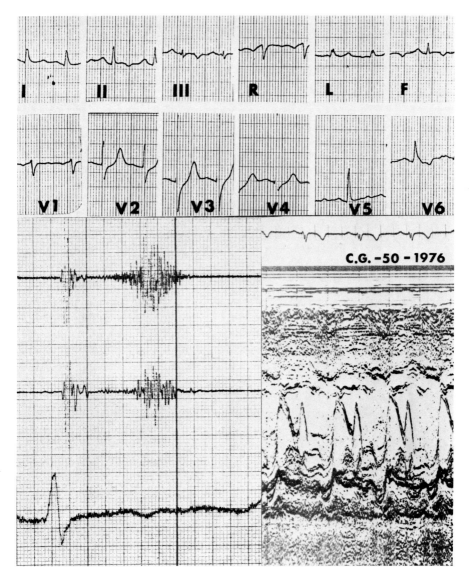

FIG. 8.3. *Case 87.* EKG in a 50-year-old woman with the chief complaint of atypical chest pain. T wave inversion in the inferior leads and in V_6 and tall T waves in V_2 and V_3 are seen. Phonocardiogram shows a late systolic murmur. Sixteen years earlier, a midsystolic click and a late systolic murmur were recorded. Echocardiogram shows midsystolic dipping (*arrow*).

et al.'s survey (233). The latter study mentioned the additional presence of "junctional ST segment changes" in 35% of their patients.

In summary, T wave inversion with or without minimal ST depression occurs in about one-third of patients with MVP seen by cardiologists. These ab-

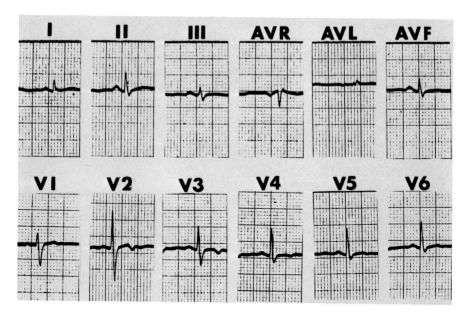

FIG. 8.4. Case 84. T wave inversion in the right precordial leads in a 46-year-old woman with idiopathic MVP and normal coronary arteriogram. T waves are flat in the inferior and left precordial leads.

normalities are characteristically noted in the inferior leads with frequent additional involvement of the left precordial leads. However, the right precordial leads may exhibit similar changes albeit in a relatively small number of patients. The T wave inversion may be diffuse (276,334).

The ST -T changes in this syndrome may occur on standing (71,165,302) or on exercise (326). They may be induced by hyperventilation and standing as shown by Jacobs et al. (165) in four patients with MVP and normal basal EKG. Normalization or marked improvement of the ST -T changes was induced by the oral administration of 20 mg propranolol in 28 of 35 patients studied by Abinader (1). This author postulated "an autonomic imbalance resulting in sympathetic overactivity" in MVP and recommended that the propranolol test be used to differentiate ischemic ST -T changes from those encountered in the MVP syndrome. I do not believe, however, that such generalization is warranted in the absence of a similar study in patients with proven coronary artery disease. It is possible that the decreased oxygen demand produced by beta-adrenergic blockade may normalize or improve truly ischemic T waves in some patients with coronary artery disease. Normalization of ST -T changes with beta blocking agents has also been reported in 10 patients with neurocirculatory asthenia (390), but these patients, who were not evaluated by auscultation or by echocardiography, may have had MVP (394).

Peaked T waves in the midprecordial leads have been described (18) but were noted in only seven of our first 100 patients (175). Prominent U waves were observed by Barlow and associates (18) but were uncommon in our series, occurring in four out of 100 patients (175).

EFFECT OF AMYL NITRITE ON THE EKG IN MVP (FIGS. 8.5 AND 8.6)

Dr. Joseph P. Liss and I (175) investigated the effect of amyl nitrite inhalation on the normal EKG in 19 patients with idiopathic MVP, in seven with rheumatic mitral regurgitation, and in five normal subjects. No ST -T changes occurred in the control group. In the rheumatic group, flattening of the T waves was observed in only two patients. In the MVP group, ST depression and T wave inversion in leads II, III, and AVF were noted in 12, flattening of

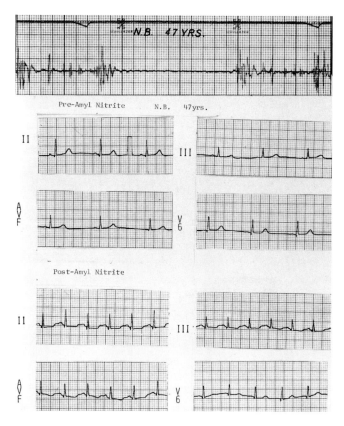

FIG. 8.5. *Case 92.* Multiple clicks and amyl nitrite (AN) test in a 47-year-old woman. A. Apex phono: multiple clicks. B. Leads II, III, and AVF show no abnormalities before AN inhalation. ST depression and T inversion in II, III, and AVF are evident after AN inhalation (heart rate 115 beats/min). (From ref. 175. By permission)

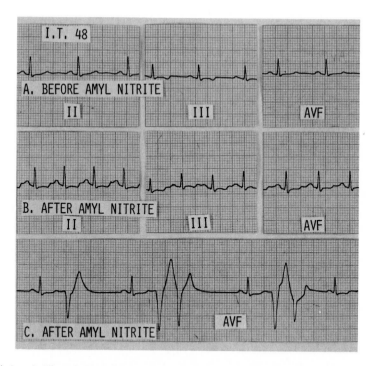

FIG. 8.6. *Case 8.* Effect of AN inhalation on the ECG in a 48-year-old woman. ST depression and T-wave inversion are noted in leads II and AVF after AN inhalation (B) Heart rate was 125 beats/min. Multiple PVCs are evident in (C). See Fig. 6.4 for phonocardiogram. (From ref. 175. By permission)

the T waves in another five, and no changes in two. Of special interest was the occurrence of T inversion in the inferior leads in two patients with "silent" prolapse. In the MVP syndrome, the lack of response usually occurred in patients whose heart rate did not rise above 105 beats/min. Full patient cooperation and adequate heart rate response are a prerequisite for a positive amyl nitrite test in MVP. This provocative maneuver may help confirm the diagnosis of idiopathic MVP when the click is inconstantly heard, in patients with "silent" MVP, and in patients with MVP, pansystolic murmur and no clicks who have been erroneously labeled as rheumatic. We postulated that amyl nitrite decreases afterload, left ventricular end-diastolic and systolic volume, and thus increases MVP and retraction on the papillary muscle (48). This latter effect produces ischemia as expressed by ST-T changes. The ST-T changes produced by amyl nitrite are not helpful in differentiating idiopathic MVP from coronary artery disease because similar changes have been reported in the latter (190). The increased contractility, the tachycardia, and abbreviation of diastole, as well as the acute reduction of coronary perfusion pressure that follows exposure to this drug, are probably responsible for the ischemic ST -T changes in coronary artery disease.

The specificity of the amyl nitrite EKG test in the differential diagnosis of MVP in the absence of coronary artery disease requires further investigation, because T wave inversion was reported in 15 of 100 young pilots, ranging in age from 17 to 25 years, and exhibiting no abnormal cardiac signs. (256). However, these 15 pilots were not evaluated for MVP.

"EVANESCENT" T WAVES IN MVP

Variability of the T waves with occasional normalization was noted in a few series (18,345) and was evident in 13 of our 42 patients (175) (Fig. 8.7), leading occasionally to the diagnosis of acute coronary episodes (169). Because of the association of chest pain and changing ST -T segments, coronary artery disease was suspected in 20 of these patients, who were subsequently shown to have a normal coronary arteriogram. In a few of these patients with severe chest pain at rest, unstable angina was suspected (380).

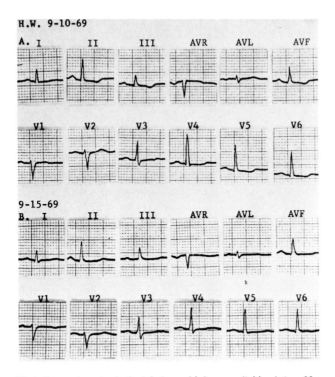

FIG. 8.7. Case 32. A. T wave inversion in the inferior and left precordial leads in a 32-year-old woman with "silent" MVP and normal coronary arteriogram. B. Six days later, the T waves are only flattened. (From ref. 175. By permission)

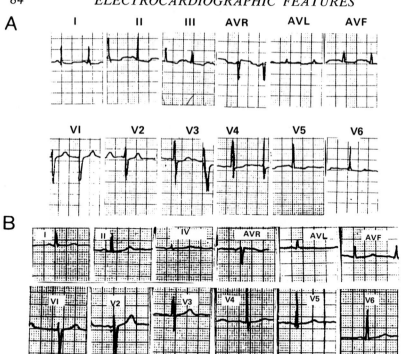

FIG. 8.8. *Case 190.* Electrocardiograms in a 32-year-old woman with severe chest pain, "silent" MVP, and normal coronary arteriogram, showing variability in T waves, probably due to heart rate. The repolarization abnormalities were not related to chest pain. A. Repolarization abnormalities in inferior and left precordial leads. Heart rate was 115 beats/min. B. EKG taken one day later shows normalization of the T waves. Heart rate was 79 beats/min. (See Fig. 6.12 for left cineventriculogram).

In patients with evanescent T waves, heart rate was the common denominator associated with EKG abnormalities (Figs. 8.8–8.10). An increase in heart rate, usually in the range of 100 beats/min is, in my opinion, the mechanism responsible for the occurrence of ST -T abnormalities in MVP patients who have a normal baseline EKG. The tachycardia may occur spontaneously, or may be induced by emotional tension, exercise, hyperventilation and amyl nitrite inhalation, and so forth. It results in a small left ventricular volume with an increase in prolapse leading to increased traction on the papillary muscle and ischemia. The decreased left ventricular volume in the standing position is due not only to associated tachycardia but also to peripheral venous pooling. Normalization of the EKG with beta-adrenergic blockage is probably due to slowing of the heart rate and to decreased contractility resulting in larger left ventricular volume (1).

The increased heart rate may not be the only factor responsible for transient T wave changes in MVP. Barlow and Pocock(19) published an EKG tracing in a 28-year-old man "whose Holter monitoring showed several episodes of progressive T wave inversion with return to normality, unrelated to any specific activity or to emotion."

QT INTERVAL IN IDIOPATHIC MVP

Prolongation of the QT interval in this syndrome has been reported (98,143,154,332). This finding could not be confirmed by Barlow and Pocock (19) who analyzed the EKG of 144 patients and found that only one, a 38-year-old woman, had a slightly prolonged QTc (0.47 sec). Swartz et al. (355) compiled data on 589 patients with MVP and arrhythmias from the literature and found prolonged QT interval in 44 (7.5%). The QT interval was reported in only 94 patients and was found prolonged in 44 (47%). I have not carried out an extensive analysis of the QT interval in this syndrome, but I have been impressed by the normalcy of the QT interval in the patients whom I have studied.

In view of these contradictory reports, I believe that the prevalence and significance of the QT prolongation in MVP merits further investigation.

ABNORMALITIES OF THE QRS IN MVP

Anterior and inferior myocardial infarction patterns have been reported in this syndrome. Tuqan et al. (366) recently reported on two young women, aged 32 and 36 years respectively, with midsystolic clicks and electrocardio-graphic and vectorcardiographic evidence of transmural anterior myocardial infarction, in the absence of a clinical history of myocardial infarction and in association with normal coronary arteriograms. The same authors were able to collect six other cases (18,222,226,385) with the MVP syndrome and Q waves that were either suggestive or diagnostic of transmural myocardial in-farction. In five of these patients, the infarct pattern was diaphragmatic and a normal coronary arterigram was described in three of the six. Subsequently, Chesler et al. (70) published their findings in four young patients with MVP who presented with clinical evidence of acute myocardial infarction, unlike the eight patients just mentioned, whose EKG provided the only suggestion of myocardial infarction. It is possible that these eight patients may have had "a silent infarction" or that the abnormal Q waves were not actually indicative of a true infarction. More cases should be studied before the significance of these cases becomes clear. There is always a possibility that we are dealing with casual association of idiopathic MVP and myocardial infarction with nor-mal coronary arteries, an entity whose etiology has not been elucidated. (See Chap. 4 for further discussion).

ARRHYTHMIAS IN IDIOPATHIC MVP

Ventricular and atrial arrhythmias are probably the most common manifestations of this syndrome (19,98,108,175,355) (Figs. 8.11A, 8.11B, and 8.12). A wide variety of arrhythmias has been encountered but premature ventricular contractions (PVCs) are the most prevalent rhythm disturbances.

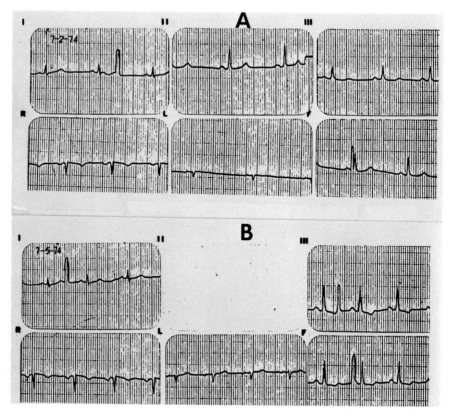

FIG. 8.9. *Case 197.* Electrocardiogram in a 46-year-old man with severe chest pain, "silent" MVP, and normal coronary arteriogram. Note variability of T waves, during hospitalization probably due to heart rate. The repolarization abnormalities were not related to chest pain. A. No repolarization abnormalities. Heart rate was 66 beats/min. B. T wave inversion in III. Initial T inversion in AVF. Heart rate was 87 beats/min.

Ventricular Arrhythmias

PVCs were encountered in 25 of our first 100 patients, on standard rest EKGs (175). A much higher prevalence was documented by Holter dynamic electrocardiography and by exercise tests. Kreisman et al. (205) were probably the first to use, in this syndrome, 24-hr Holter monitoring, the most sensitive method of study of arrhythmias: all of their 10 patients displayed multifocal PVCs. Criley and Kissel (84) also monitored 22 patients by means of the Holter technique and reported PVCs in 17, premature atrial contractions in 13, and paroxysmal atrial tachycardia in 13. Using the same technique, DeMaria et al. (98) observed PVCs in 58% of their 31 patients. A higher prevalence of 75% was reported by Winkle et al. (384) in 24 patients and by Campbell et al. (52) in 20 patients. Swartz et al. (355) reviewed all cases (a total of 589 patients) of the association of MVP and arrhythmias published in the English language literature. The average age of these patients

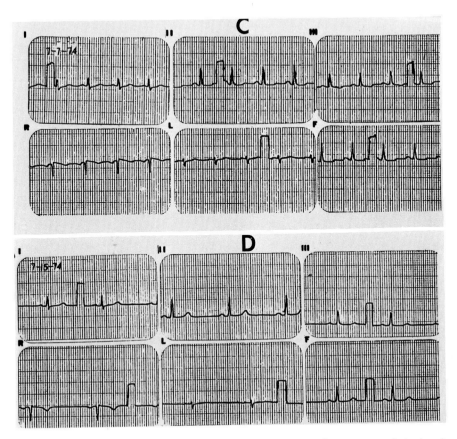

FIG. 8.9.C. T wave inversion in inferior leads. Heart rate was 105 beats/min. D. No repolarization abnormalities. Heart rate was 57 beats/min. (See Fig. 12.10 for left cineventriculogram).

was 37.8 years. The sex was indicated in 448 patients, 308 (69.8%) of whom were women. Most of these patients were symptomatic: of the 423 whose symptoms were included 44.3% had palpitations, 11.6% had light-headedness, and 4% had syncope. PVCs were found in 55% of these 589 patients, and ventricular tachycardia was documented in 6.3%. Episodes of ventricular tachycardia ranged from one to more than 20 attacks in a 24-hr period.

The significance of ventricular arrhythmias noted on 24-hr Holter monitoring and exercise was evaluated by Winkle et al. (384) in 24 patients showing echocardiographic prolapse and not specifically selected for presence or absence of arrhythmias. They described two subsets of patients. Approximately one-half of their patients showed more than one PVC on the treadmill test and frequent (more than 425) PVCs on Holter monitor; the majority of these patients had complex ventricular arrhythmias including ventricular tachycardia in six patients. The other half showed none or only one PVC on treadmill testing and infrequent (fewer than 50) PVCs on the 24-hr ambulatory EKG; this

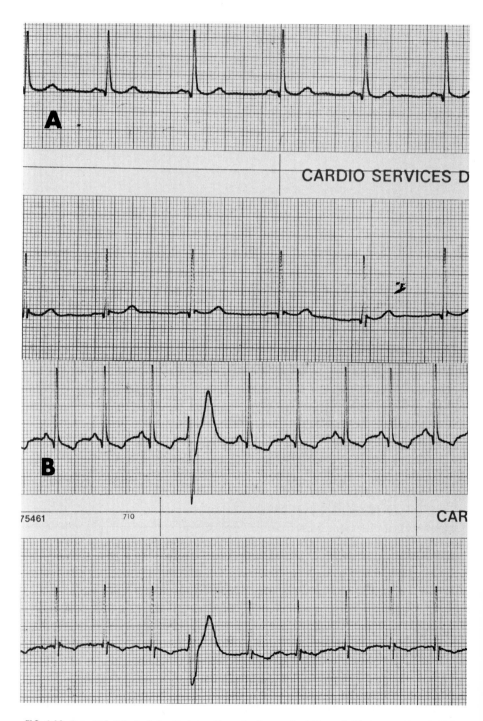

CARDIO SERVICES D

75461   710   CAR

FIG. 8.10. *Case 331.* Effect of sinus tachycardia on the T wave in a 30-year-old woman with midsystolic click, in the course of a 24-hr Holter monitoring (2 channels). A. Upright T waves. Sinus rate was 65/min B. Inverted T waves at rest. Sinus rate was 107.1 PVC. See Fig. 8.12.

group had almost no complex ventricular arrhythmias and their PVC frequency was felt to "come close to the number of PVCs per 24 hr that one can consider as normal" (283). It was noted, in this interesting study, that 58% of the patients with frequent PVCs showed a statistically significant reduction of PVCs during sleep and 17% showed an increase. A general lack of correlation between symptoms and recorded arrhythmias was well documented in this study: patients were generally unaware of the recorded arrhythmias or complained of palpitations when the monitor showed no rhythm disturbance. We have noted this symptom– arrhythmia discordance –in several of our patients (Fig. 8.12). In two of these patients with frequent palpitations, we used a Cardio-Beeper (manufactured by Survival Technology Inc.) for frequent transtelephone transmission of EKG tracings for 1 to 2 weeks and have been impressed by the absence of arrhythmias including sinus tachycardia during palpitations and, conversely, by the frequent occurrence of nonsensed arrhythmias. Winkle et al. (384) found the 24-hr ambulatory EKG to be more sensitive than the treadmill test and both were superior to the 12 lead ECG for detecting arrhythmias in MVP.

Malignant ventricular arrhythmias (e.g., ventricular tachycardia and fibrillation) (53,228,386) occur in a small number of patients with MVP and will be discussed in Chap. 14.

Supraventricular Arrhythmias

Supraventricular arrhythmias that were infrequent in some series reporting standard electrocardiographic studies (154,175,211) were more common in those based on dynamic electrocardiography: 35% (98) and 64% (384) respectively. In one series (384) 15 of 24 patients studied demonstrated atrial premature contractions, and complex atrial arrhythmias were found among patients with infrequent as well as with frequent premature atrial contractions. Supraventricular tachycardia was detected in seven of these patients. In 22 patients reviewed by Criley and Kissel (84), 15 had PACs and six had paroxysmal atrial tachycardia.

The atrial arrhythmias in this syndrome include paroxysmal atrial tachycardia, atrial flutter, and fibrillation (19,108,321). I was impressed by the occurrence of symptomatic sinus tachycardia unrelated to physical activity or to emotional stress. This arrhythmia that was documented on Holter monitoring in six of our patients with a sinus rate reaching 140–150 beats/min may represent a sinus node reentrant tachycardia. The patients complained of palpitations, generalized weakness, dizziness, and near fainting during these episodes.

Relationship of Arrhythmias to Clinical and Electrocardiographic Features in MVP

DeMaria et al. (98) found no relation between arrhythmias to either ST segment or T wave abnormalities or to prolongation of the QT interval. Moreover,

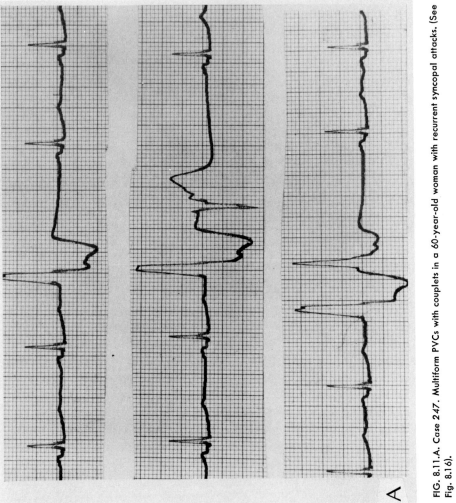

FIG. 8.11.A. Case 247. Multiform PVCs with couplets in a 60-year-old woman with recurrent syncopal attacks. (See Fig. 8.16).

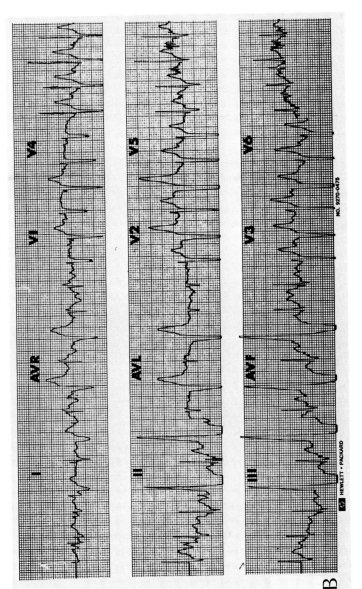

FIG. 8.11.B. Ventricular bigeminy induced by exercise in a 25-year-old man with MVP.

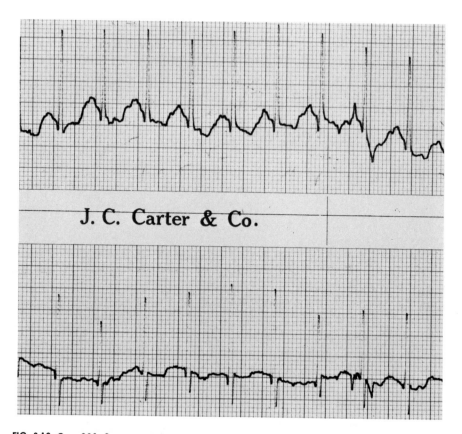

FIG. 8.12. *Case 331.* Supraventricular tachycardia at a rate of 148/min in a 30-year-old woman with midsystolic click, in the course of a 24-hr Holter monitoring (2 channels). The tachycardia (probably sinus in origin) was not sensed by the patient. Note T wave inversion. (See Fig. 8.10).

no correlation could be found regarding sex, age, severity of MVP, or of mitral regurgitation. However, a more recent study (53), dealing with 20 patients with MVP and using Holter monitoring, described a higher incidence of serious ventricular arrhythmias (ventricular tachycardia and fibrillation) in patients with inferolateral ST and T wave abnormalities. In a review of sudden death in MVP (384), there were six patients in whom EKG had been reported and six of these patients showed ST -T abnormalities. Further studies are needed to correlate ST -T changes with the incidence and severity of arrhythmias and to determine their usefulness in identifying those patients at risk for sudden death.

Bradyarrhythmias and Conduction Defects

Bradyarrhythmias and conduction defects have been reported in this syndrome but have been relatively rare (19,108,175,276,355). Winkle et al.

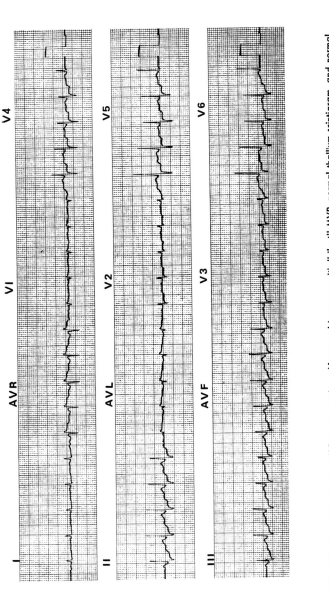

FIG. 8.13. Case 326. Positive EKG stress test in a 61-year-old woman with "silent" MVP, normal thallium scintigram, and normal coronary arteriogram (Case 5 in Table 8.1). A 2 mm ST segment depression is noted. (Courtesy of Dr. Joseph P. Liss)

(384) reported no bradyarrhythmias in their ambulatory EKG study of 24 patients with MVP. First degree AV block occurs in about 3% of patients in two series (19,108) but this conduction abnormality is not uncommon in the general population. Right bundle branch block, left bundle branch block, and particularly left anterior hemiblock have been reported but are less common (19,145,175,180,302,370,371). In our series of 350 patients, left bundle branch block was noted in two patients, right bundle branch block in two, and left anterior fascicular block in two.

Two patients described by Gulotta (149) had permanent pacemakers implanted because of recurrent syncopal episodes that appeared related to the development of complete AV block in one patient. One of these patients was studied with His bundle electrocardiography and prolonged HV interval with intermittent second degree heart block was demonstrated with the block proximal to the His bundle.

A few recent reports (98,217) documented a surprising frequency of bradyarrhythmia and conduction defects in this syndrome. In one series (98) of 31 patients with MVP, Holter monitoring revealed bradyarrhythmia in nine (29%): two had sinus bradycardia, six marked sinus arrhythmias, two periods of sinoatrial arrest, and two wandering atrial pacemakers. In another series (217) 11 members of a family with a high prevalence of MVP and bradycardia were investigated. Three patients with both MVP and bradycardia had recurrent syncope. Atrial pacing studies documented a marked prolongation of atrial– His interval and inability to maintain a 1:1 atrioventricular conduction when paced at a rate of 120 beats/min. SA and AV nodal dysfunction was documented. The authors presented evidence favoring joint transmission of MVP and bradycardia as an autosomal dominant trait. Syncope resulting from bradycardia was successfully treated by pacemaker placement in two patients. As indicated by these authors, there have been no embryologic, anatomic, or physiological studies of the relation between the conduction system and valvular abnormalities. SA nodal disease was also described in a third series (398) that reported on Holter monitoring in six patients with all six showing marked sinus arrhythmia and three of these showing sinoatrial Wenckebach patterns. In a fourth series (321) of 27 patients, 10 patients demonstrated conduction defects: two had 2:1 block at the AV node, one had left anterior fascicular block, one left anterior fascicular block and prolonged PR interval, one right bundle branch block and left anterior fascicular block, one right bundle branch block, and two left bundle branch block with one complete heart block.

Other case reports of MVP associated with AV and SA node abnormalities were recently published (49,103,234,359,392). Martin (234) reported on a 68-year-old woman with midsystolic click, late systolic murmur, normal coronary arteriogram, angiographic MVP, and transient complete heart block associated with "a feeling of dizziness and faintness." Congenital AV block, narrow QRS, and MVP were reported in a 41-year-old woman (359): the block was shown to be at the AV node by His bundle recording. Another patient, a 24-year-old man with MVP and intermittent complete AV block masquerading as epilepsy was reported by Woodly et al. (392); the patient's symptoms were all totally corrected by implantation of an epicardial demand pacemaker. DeSilva and Shubrooks (103) reported a 20-year-old male with MVP, sinus bradycardia with marked sinus arrhythmias, and high grade AV block probably with onset in infancy; there was a lack of relationship of symptoms of lightheadedness and near syncope to any rhythm disturbances and electrophysiological studies demonstrated the site of block to be proximal to the His bundle. Finally, a case of MVP, right bundle branch block and left anterior hemiblock in a patient with Ehler–Danlos syndrome was recently reported (49).

In conclusion, bradyarrhythmias are not infrequently associated with MVP. Sinoatrial nodal abnormalities (sinus bradycardia, SA node block, pronounced sinus arrhythmias) are the most common bradyarrhythmias in this syndrome, but are also common in the normal population (see below). AV nodal abnormalities and conduction defects in the His bundle and its branches are uncommon in MVP and may represent a chance association. Altogether, complete heart block has been reported in only six patients with MVP (149,234,321, 359,392). To the best of my knowledge, studies of the sinus node arterial supply similar to those carried out by James (167) on Marfan's syndrome have not been performed on MVP. This author has described medial degeneration and hyperplasia as well as intimal proliferation of the small coronary vessels supplying the sinus and atrioventricular nodes in Marfan's syndrome and these abnormalities should be sought in MVP. The possibility of involvement of the cardiac conduction system by the myxomatous process should be investigated. Shappell et al. (332), who studied the conduction system in a patient with MVP and QT interval prolongation who died suddenly, have reported no abnormalities.

Preexcitation in MVP

An association between preexcitation and MVP was noted for the first time by Gallagher et al. (133). Out of 68 patients with WPW, seven had a midsystolic click with or without an apical murmur and MVP was documented by echocardiography, left ventriculography, or both. The same group (135) subsequently reviewed a larger experience with the preexcitation syndrome and noted the presence of MVP (documented by echocardiography, left ventriculography or both) in 10 patients. A higher prevalence was reported by Teichholz and Taegtmeyer (358) in 16 patients with preexcitation, six of whom (38%) had MVP by echocardiography. Five of these patients had a midsystolic click and/or late systolic murmur. This association has also been reported by other investigators (33,51,108,183,207,231).

In our series of 350 patients, we observed preexcitation in only one patient.

However, a higher prevalence of preexcitation in MVP was reported by Antonelli et al. (7) who submitted 41 consecutive patients with MVP seen over a 12 month period to careful electrocardiographic studies including His bundle recording and programmed atrial stimulation if there was any suspicion of a delta wave. These authors noted preexcitation in six out of 41 examined cases (14.6%) and suggested that the "association is not an occasional one."

Bypass tracts in patients with MVP may be concealed and used only during supraventricular tachycardia as shown in a recent study of 12 patients with MVP utilizing intracardiac recording and stimulation techniques (183). Of these 12 patients, three had a short PR interval, one WPW type A, and eight normal EKGs. Six of the eight patients with normal EKGs were shown to have left sided atrioventricular bypass tracts. The authors stress the need for electrophysiological studies to diagnose these bypass tracts because surface EKGs may be misleading. They also felt that these tracts are probably related to the mitral valve since they are always left sided. Of interest is the right sided location of the bypass tracts in Ebstein's anomaly, a disease of the tricuspid valve.

In their earlier study, Gallagher et al. (133) indicated that the WPW syndrome associated with MVP was of type A. In their subsequent reports on 10 patients with MVP and WPW (135) they found the accessory pathway to be situated in the left free wall atrioventricular groove in four, and in the septal region in three; in the remaining three patients they could not ascertain with certainty whether the pathway was located in the septal region or in the left atrioventricular groove. The six cases reported by another group (358) were classified as follows: three with type A, two with type B and one with Lown-Ganong-Levine syndrome. Likewise, in a recent series (7), both right and left sided accessory pathways were reported.

In an interesting case of MVP associated with intermittent WPW (33), the click was recorded only during preexcitation, suggesting an abnormal ventricular activation pattern as the cause of the MVP. However, in an echocardiographic study (358) one patient with intermittent WPW type A had MVP during both preexcitation and normal conduction. The latter finding would suggest that MVP in preexcitation "is not secondary to an abnormal activation pattern of the left ventricle and papillary muscles but rather to an associated structural abnormality of the mitral valve" (358). I am inclined to agree with this statement and to explain the findings of the former case (33) as possibly due to variation of left ventricular volume occurring as follows: during preexcitation in type A WPW the early activation and contraction of the posterior left ventricular wall presents a smaller left ventricular volume when subsequent normal activation and contraction occurs, allowing more pronounced excursion of the mitral leaflets and permitting the left ventricular volume to reach the critical click volume (242); in the absence of preexcitation in this case it is possible that the left ventricular systolic volume never reached the critical size needed to induce a click. It is possible that the association of MVP and preexcitation may be due to the defective dilated and myxomatous mitral annulus in MVP that allows persistent muscular bridges between the atrium and the ventricle.

True Prevalence and Significance of ST-T Changes and Arrhythmias in MVP

Judging from the several reports just mentioned, most investigators concluded that ventricular and atrial arrhythmias are common in idiopathic MVP. In one series of 31 patients who had MVP (98) only 16% had no arrhythmia during ambulatory monitoring. Significantly, less arrhythmias occurred in 40 normal subjects during monitoring: 58% PVCs in MVP versus 25% in "normal" subjects. Since the latter group underwent invasive studies for "evaluation of chest pain," the 25% prevalence of PVCs in this group may be higher than in the normal population. Conversely, the prevalence of arrhythmias in the MVP group may be higher than in an unselected MVP group, since this study, as well as others having originated from cardiac referral centers may have overestimated the frequency of arrhythmias "by virtue of sampling errors" (219). For these surveys to be meaningful as far as prevalence of arrhythmias in normal subjects and in unscreened subjects with MVP, they should be based on ambulatory monitoring in these two groups. To my knowledge, no such studies have been carried out. Procacci et al.'s (286) study revealed arrhythmias in five of 74 women (7%) found to have MVP out of 1,169 women examined: two patients had occasional PVCs, one had frequent PVCs and a short run of ventricular tachycardia. In this survey, dependent wives of Airforce personnel were urged to report for a physical examination as part of a "Women's Health Week" and were described by the authors as a group who considered itself healthy. It is possible that symptomatic patients who may have had MVP with or without clicks and murmurs did not report for physical examination because they already knew that they had heart disease. Therefore in this survey (286), the prevalence of arrhythmias may have been underestimated. Moreover, no ambulatory EKG monitoring was carried out and the 7% prevalence rate of arrhythmia may be misleading because of the known lack of sensitivity of resting EKG in detecting arrhythmias. In a second survey (233) of 100 healthy females, ambulatory monitoring was carried out in 31 and revealed a 60% prevalence of arrhythmias in 10 women with auscultatory and echocardiographic MVP versus 28.6% in eight women without MVP and none in 13 women with either echocardiographic or phonocardiographic evidence of MVP. The authors felt that the number of Holter electrocardiographic recordings was too small for statistical comparison among the three groups.

The prevalence of ST -T changes in these epidemiologic surveys was 15% in

Procacci et al.'s (286) 76 patients but EKGs were not taken in the subjects without proven MVP. In Markiewicz et al.'s (233) survey the difference between the two groups with MVP and without MVP regarding the incidence of ST -T wave abnormalities was not statistically different.

The available information on the true prevalence of arrhythmias and ST -T changes in MVP has remained incomplete and often contradictory. To answer those critics who feel that the occurrence of these abnormalities is not higher in MVP than in the general population, further epidemiologic studies are needed. The prevalence of MVP should be established in a completely unscreened population group. Subjects with proven MVP and the control group should have rest and ambulatory EKG studies.

Arrhythmias in the normal population were studied by Brodsky et al. (41) by 24-hr continuous EKG monitoring in 50 male medical students: 25 (50%) exhibited PVCs but only one (2%) had more than 50 such contractions in 24 hr. The authors concluded that frequent atrial and ventricular contractions are unusual in a young adult population but that bradyarrhythmias (including marked sinus arrhythmia with sinus pauses, sinus bradycardia and nocturnal type I second degree AV block) are common. No such studies have been carried out in a normal female population. This study would suggest that the normal population does not demonstrate the high prevalence and frequency of ventricular arrhythmia noted in MVP. However, the prevalence of bradyarrhythmia in the normal population casts doubt on the pathological significance of this type of arrhythmia when noted in MVP.

To evaluate the significance of the ST -T changes seen on routine electrocardiography, as an indication of MVP particularly in young and middle aged females, a group of patients with these findings should be evaluated for MVP by auscultation and echocardiography and compared to a control group with normal EKGs.

From the available information, I believe that future studies would confirm a significantly higher prevalence of arrhythmias in patients with MVP than in control groups. In view of the relatively common occurrence of "silent MVP" I concur with DeMaria et al.'s (98) statement that echocardiography is advisable in patients, particularly young women, with unexplained arrhythmias.

Mechanism of ST -T Abnormalities and Arrhythmias in MVP

To explain the genesis of various electrocardiographic and rhythm abnormalities in MVP, several theories have been proposed. Proponents of the myocardial theory have postulated a focal cardiomyopathy (149,322). Excessive traction on the papillary muscles by the prolapsed leaflets has been advocated as a logical explanation by proponents of the valvular theory (73,169,175, 276). This excessive traction interferes with the blood supply or induces spasm of the small coronary arteries (71). To add further credence to the theory, Cobbs and King (73) carried out epicardial mapping of the PVCs during mitral valve replacement in one of their patients and were able to localize earliest epicardial breakthrough to an area over the site of the posterior papillary muscle. Another factor responsible for ventricular arrhythmia may be mechanical stimulation of the endocardium by the chordae (336). Arrhythmias may also originate from the endocardial friction lesions and their myocardial extension (317). The abnormally tense mitral leaflets that contain muscle fibers capable of developing diastolic depolarization (389) may be another source of arrhythmias in MVP. Observations by Witt and Cranefield (388) in the simian mitral valve suggest that mitral valve fibers generate slow response action potentials, that triggerable sustained rhythmic activity may be a property of this slow response and "that such activity may cause the types of cardiac arrhythmias that usually are attributed to re-entry." Criley et al. (86) proposed a mechanical theory postulating that during early diastole the leaflets that are above the level of the mitral annulus abruptly dump the blood contained within their ventricular aspects into the base of the left ventricle (diastolic dumping). Although Criley's hypothesis and the papillary traction theory do not explain the intermittent nature of the arrhythmias, hemodynamic changes resulting in variation in left ventricular geometry and volume may account for this sporadic occurrence (355).

The nature of ventriculary arrhythmias in MVP has not been fully explored by the newer electrophysiologic techniques to determine if a reentrant mechanism is present. Wellens et al. (377) studied three patients with MVP and ventricular tachycardia. In one of their patients tachycardia could be reproduced by two successive ventricular extra stimuli (S_1,S_2,S_3 extra stimulation), indicating a reentrant mechanism. However, in two other patients there was failure to initiate the tachycardia.

The relatively frequent association of MVP and preexcitation provides a mechanism for supraventricular tachycardia in MVP. Kastor and Josephson (183) studied 12 patients with MVP and supraventricular tachycardia by means of His bundle electrogram, atrial endocardial mapping, and programmed atrial stimulation. In only five of their patients, an AV nodal reentrant tachycardia was demonstrated; in the remaining seven an atrioventricular accessory pathway formed one limb of the reentrant circuit. The prevalence of bypass tract participation in supraventricular tachycardia was, therefore, inordinately high. In the authors' experience, AV nodal reentry is the mechanism in two-thirds of the episodes of supraventricular tachycardia in the general population while bypass grafts are operative in only 20% of cases. This study suggests that bypass tracts are common in MVP and play an important role in the genesis of supraventricular tachycardia in this disorder. Camous et al. (51) reported the case of a 36-year-old patient with MVP, preexcitation through a left atrioventricular pathway, and attacks of tachycardia at a rate of 180 to 340 associated with presyncope.

The mechanism of the arrhythmias in this syndrome is probably multifactorial. I would favor traction on the papillary muscle as the mechanism for the ST -T abnormalities and arrhythmias. Further studies are clearly needed to elucidate the mechanism of the arrhythmias in this syndrome and "to determine which of the possible mechanisms is the most important" (355).

STRESS STUDIES IN MVP

Studies have been carried out to determine the effect of exercise on chest pain in this syndrome and its differentiation from angina pectoris. The exercise test has also been utilized for the unmasking of arrhythmias (Fig. 8.11B). In earlier studies, abnormal post exercise EKG was noted in this syndrome (95,162,385) despite a normal coronary arteriogram (Fig. 8.13). However, Gooch et al. (144) could not duplicate these findings. The stress test that appears to unmask ventricular irritability (144,275,385) was recommended in all patients with this syndrome with a view to antiarrhythmic therapy (275).

Because of increasing interest in this syndrome, several investigators reevaluated the role of exercise in the diagnosis of MVP and the detection and management of arrhythmias associated with it. In MVP with normal coronary arteriogram, exercise was reported in inducing ST -T changes often indistinguishable from those observed in coronary artery disease (19,137,165,231, 240,264,283). In a recent study (240) of 25 patients with confirmed MVP (19 with normal coronary arteriograms and six with associated coronary artery disease), stress EKGs were not helpful in diagnosing associated coronary artery disease because of high incidence (10 of 19 or 53%) of false positive tests in idiopathic MVP. The stress test had only a 48% overall accuracy. The presence or absence of chest pain during exercise was not helpful since nine of 19 patients with normal coronary arteriograms experienced pain. "Ischemic" ST -T changes have also been observed in children (326): during exercise ST depression of 1–3 mm occurred in three of ten males with MVP as compared to four of 55 controls and in nine of 20 females as compared to seven of 48 controls, a statistically significant difference.

On the basis of these data and on my own experience, I do not believe that exercise induced ST-T changes should be used to differentiate idiopathic MVP from coronary artery disease when evaluating a patient with chest pain.

The thallium 201 stress test is helpful in this differential diagnosis, despite two recent abstracts (248,268) that reported abnormal thallium exercise tests in patients with idiopathic MVP and normal coronary arteriogram, prompting one group (248) to state that in patients with MVP this test "cannot be used to detect or exclude coronary artery disease." Indeed, a third abstract (198) found that MVP was not associated with regional myocardial ischemia as depicted by stress myocardial scintigraphy. The usefulness of myocardial perfusion scintigraphy and its advantage over stress electrocardiography was well documented in a recent study by Massie et al. (240) who reported that all 19 patients with MVP and normal coronary arteriogram had normal thallium

201 exercise scintigram "indicating that the radionuclide technique is highly specific of the diagnosis of coronary artery disease in these subjects," and that, conversely, each of the six patients with MVP and coronary artery disease had segmental perfusion defects. The authors rightfully pointed out that their findings do not exclude ischemia as a cause for symptoms and EKG abnormalities in MVP because an ischemic zone could be focal and too small to be detected by the technique or could be generalized and, therefore, undetectable. Our experience with thallium scintigraphy is summarized in Table 8.1. None of a group of six patients with idiopathic MVP showed perfusion defects on thallium 201 myocardial scintigraphy (Figs. 8.14 and 8.15).

Further studies are needed to elucidate the diagnostic value of stress scintigraphy in MVP, and to confirm our findings and that of others (198,240).

Friesinger et al. (132) described a group of 40 patients who had "ischemic" electrocardiographic response to exercise but who did not fulfill the usual criteria for ischemic heart disease. These patients developed an unusual increase in heart rate and ST segment changes on standing, and "ischemic" EKG changes unaccompanied by chest discomfort occurring early in exercise and disappearing as exercise proceeded. The authors ascribed these changes to vasoregulatory abnormalities. However, since echocardiographic studies were not performed, it is possible that this group included a high percentage of patients with MVP. This possibility was confirmed by Jacobs et al. (165) who studied 11 patients including eight women with similar EKG findings, and with normal coronary arteriograms in five and no coronary artery disease by clinical criteria in six, and who found that four had MVP by auscultation or left ventriculography. These ST -T changes were also induced by the orthostatic position and by hyperventilation. The authors stated that "it is interesting that the 11 patients with false positive ischemic ST -T changes on hyperventilation had significantly higher heart rate than the 17 patients with proven coronary artery disease and no ischemic changes on hyperventilation." The occurrence of ST -T changes in the upright position and hyperventilation and the probable relationship of tachycardia, decreased left ventricular volume, and increase in MVP with increased traction on the papillary muscle were discussed earlier in this chapter. The occurrence of ST depression on standing and hyperventilation with normalization as the stress test proceeds may constitute findings pointing to MVP as a diagnostic possibility. In one study (230) severe ST depression occurred almost only in the post exercise period, but further investigation is needed to confirm the diagnostic value of this finding.

Various arrhythmias have been induced by exercise in patients with MVP but a 24-hr ambulatory EKG has been found more sensitive than the treadmill test for detecting arrhythmia in this syndrome (384). Yet the clinical usefulness of the stress test should not be underestimated (275,384) in unmasking significant arrhythmia in this syndrome, and in providing objective data in support of antiarrhythmic therapy.

Brown et al. (42) investigated the effect of inflight maneuvers involving high

TABLE 8.1. Thallium-201 myocardial perfusion studies, following stress testing in six patients with idiopathic MVP

Patient (no. and initials)	Sex	Age	Auscultation	Echocardiogram	Stress EKG	Left ventriculography	Coronary arteriography	Thallium
1. A.T.	F	60	early click	TU	Negative	MVP	Normal	Negative
2. L.S.	F	29	LSM	MVP	Positive	MVP	Normal	Negative
3. E.H.	F	27	MSC	normal	Negative	MVP	Normal	Negative
4. G.A.	M	60	MSC-LSM	NP	Negative	NP	NP	Negative
5. M.B.	F	61	"Silent" MVP	NP	Positive	MVP	Normal	Negative
6. B.G.	F	40	MSC	Suggestive of MVP	Borderline	MVP	Normal	Negative

Courtesy of Doctors Joseph P. Liss and James D. Slavin.
MSC, Midsystolic click; LSM, Late systolic murmur; TU, Technically unsatisfactory; NP, Not performed.

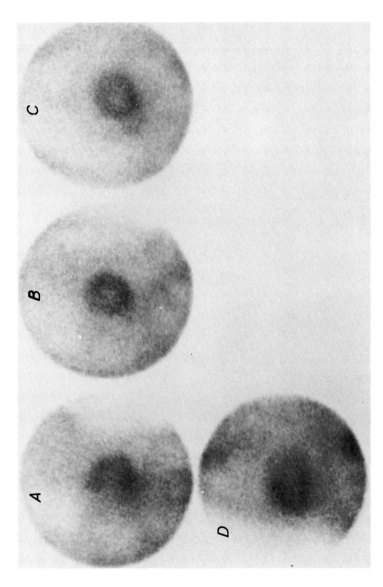

FIG. 8.14. Case 325. Normal stress thallium—201 myocardial scintigram in a 60-year-old woman with intractable chest pain, early click, MVP on left ventriculography and normal coronary arteriogram (Case 1 in Table 8.1. See Fig. 6.5 for phonocardiogram and left ventriculogram). A. Anterior view. B. 30° LAO view. C. 60° LAO view. D. Lateral view. (Courtesy of Drs. James D. Slavin and Joseph P. Liss).

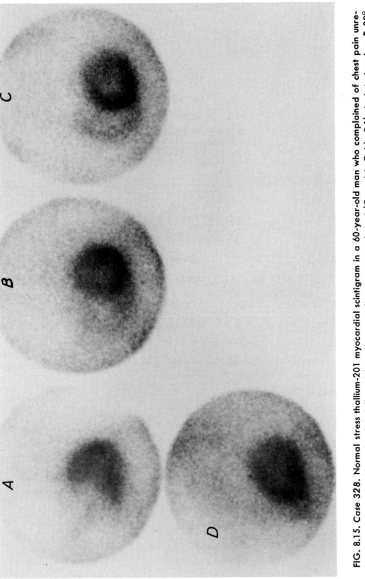

FIG. 8.15. Case 328. Normal stress thallium-201 myocardial scintigram in a 60-year-old man who complained of chest pain unrelated to activity. A midsystolic click followed by a late systolic murmur was heard (Case 4 in Table 8.1). A. Anterior view. B. 30° LAO view. C. 60° LAO view. D. Lateral view. (Courtesy of Drs. James D. Slavin and Joseph P. Liss).

$+G_2$ stress as a precipitating mechanism of arrhythmias in MVP. These maneuvers consist of a force applied to the buttocks, thighs, and/or feet in a headward direction. In two young men with a history of arrhythmias, the arrhythmias were most prominently displayed during $+G_2$ stress; one of these two cases demonstrated no rhythm disorder during or after maximal exercise stress testing. Of particular interest was the fact that these two patients developed "the first significant arrhythmias encountered in over 270 inflight hours of dynamic electrocardiography monitoring performed on a group of 90 student aviators." Left ventricular volume changes were postulated as a mechanism of the rhythm disturbances during $+G_2$ maneuvers. Another group of investigators (227) studied the arrhythmic nature of MVP in 15 otherwise healthy air crewmen (out of 989 subjects evaluated). They utilized maximal treadmill tests, 24-hr Holter monitor, orthostatic tilt table testing, and human centrifuge run. Frequent multiform PVCs and ventricular fibrillation were unmasked in two patients by this approach, necessitating their removal from flying and institution of immediate suppressive therapy.

Brown et al. (42) made the following recommendations:

1. When aviation personnel are involved, Holter monitoring, exercise testing and $+G_2$ maneuvers should be carried out for unmasking of arrhythmias.

2. While the auscultatory syndrome per se would not seem to pose a significant threat to aviation personnel, the presence of certain associated arrhythmias may serve as contraindication to a flight status.

The effect of psychological stress consisting of increasingly difficult guessing tests was investigated in 15 patients with click-murmur syndrome and 15 normal controls (76). Arrhythmias consisting of new PVCs or their increased frequency was induced in five patients but in none of the controls. Click amplitude increased in five of the 15 patients and in four, the increase was associated with arrhythmias.

Exercise Test and MVP: Summary

Exercise test in MVP may induce ST-T changes that can be similar to those observed in coronary artery disease. However, the patient with MVP frequently exhibits ST depression on standing and during hyperventilation, with normalization during exercise and pronounced abnormality after exercise. Exercise tests are less sensitive than Holter monitoring in unmasking arrhythmias in MVP but they complement the information available from rest and dynamic electrocardiography. Thallium 201 scintigraphy is probably helpful in ruling out associated coronary artery disease as a cause of repolarization abnormalities in MVP.

MANAGEMENT OF ARRHYTHMIAS IN MVP

Despite their frequency, arrhythmias in MVP are usually benign and asymptomatic. However, in a few patients, complex, repetitive, and life-threatening arrhythmias may occur, requiring aggressive management. The occurrence of sudden death, albeit rare, casts a serious omen on significant arrhythmias in this syndrome and tends to favor intervention in any decision-making process. The general experience with treatment of arrhythmias in this syndrome will be reviewed and therapeutic indications will be discussed.

Antiarrhythmic Therapy in MVP

In view of their frequency and their occasional serious nature in this syndrome, ventricular arrhythmias have been the major focus of attention. Propranolol has been advocated by most authors (19,84,144,175,264,384) as the drug of choice because, in addition to its intrinsic value as antiarrhythmic agent, it decreases left ventricular contractility, decreases heart rate, increases left ventricular volume and may, therefore, lessen the myocardial ischemia resulting from excessive traction on the papillary muscles. It may be particularly effective in exercise induced arrhythmias. It is also effective in relieving the chest pain frequently encountered in this syndrome. In those patients with MVP and prolonged QT interval and arrhythmia, propranolol has the additional benefit of shortening the QT interval. Unfortunately, it is not well tolerated by many patients with MVP because it worsens their fatigue and occasionally induces depression. In some patients, a small dosage (10 mg.q.i.d.) can be beneficial (108). The high dosage (e.g., 120–320 mg), which is generally well tolerated by patients with angina, hypertension, and arrhythmias unrelated to MVP, cannot usually be administered to patients with MVP because of side effects. Other beta-adrenergic blockers that are not available in this country may have a better tolerance level. Two of my patients who found it impossible to take propranolol because of fatigue and depression tolerated practalol well, but this drug was withdrawn by its manufacturer because of serious side effects. Bradyarrhythmias, particularly those due to sinoatrial node abnormalities, represent a contraindication to propanolol therapy. I have observed marked sinus bradycardia in MVP resulting from small doses of propranolol prompting the discontinuation of this drug. Reports of the efficacy of propranolol on arrhythmia in MVP are largely anecdotal (258). However, two groups (258,385) used dynamic electrocardiography in evaluating the antiarrhythmic effects of propranolol. One group (258) studied 10 patients using three 24-hr ambulatory EKG recordings in each patient: the first during a control period, the second 1 week after institution of a low dose propranolol therapy (80 mg daily) and the third after 2 weeks of high dose propranolol therapy (160 mg daily). In five of their patients, there was a definite reduction of more than 50% in the number of PVCs per hour, but two patients could not tolerate the higher propranolol dosage. The effect of this drug was more marked during the waking hours. The second group (385) who studied nine patients with frequent PVCs reported similar results: 75% or more reduction of PVCs in five of their patients. One of their patients had a striking increase of PVCs frequency. It is noteworthy that propranolol abolished paroxysmal ventricular tachycardia in three of four patients and the decrease in complex arrhythmias occurred in the five patients who had a reduction in PVCs frequency. Propranolol induced a significant reduction of PACs in four patients studied but did not appear to decrease the frequency of paroxysmal supraventricular tachycardia (385).

These two studies confirm the beneficial effects of propranolol. A favorable result in 50% of patients can be considered as a major accomplishment for any antiarrhythmic drug. I concur with Winkle et al. (385) that ideally "arrhythmias should be characterized before administering propranolol, the effect of therapy carefully determined, and propranolol continued only if it is effective in their treatment." Practically and for the purpose of cost effectiveness, this approach cannot be justified in a prevalent and generally benign syndrome that is frequently associated with palpitations and arrhythmias. The practicing physician, encouraged by the documentation of the antiarrhythmic efficacy of propranolol in at least 50% of patients and by its beneficial effect on chest pain, may be justified to resort empirically to this drug and to assess its results clinically. However, in the presence of serious life-threatening arrhythmias, Winkle et al.'s (385) recommendation should definitely be implemented.

Diphenylhydantoin was found effective in the management of ventricular arrhythmias by Barlow and Pocock (19). Because it shortens the QT interval, this drug has gained acceptability among those who had demonstrated prolonged QT interval in this syndrome. I have had no experience with this drug in this syndrome. However, it is a weak antiarrhythmic agent and further studies based on ambulatory monitoring and stress testing are needed to determine its usefulness in the management of arrhythmias in MVP.

Quinidine and procainamide have been used alone or in combination with propranolol (108). In the absence of prolongation of the QT interval they can be used cautiously if propranolol has been ineffective. Quinidine has been shown to have synergistic effect when added to propranolol. Demonstration of the efficacy of quinidine or procainamide by ambulatory monitoring is recommended before instituting a long term therapy with these agents. The safety and efficacy of these two drugs in MVP have not been established.

Other antiarrhythmic drugs have been recommended. Campbell et al. (53) found the orally active antiarrhythmic drug, mexiletine, effective in abolishing ventricular arrhythmias and fibrillation in four of their patients. Fasola et al. (122) administered aprindine to three patients with MVP, multiple PVCs, and recurrent ventricular tachycardia and fibrillation. Treatment with conventional antiarrhythmic agents had been tried without success in every patient before aprindine therapy was instituted. In each of the three patients, aprindine induced a marked drop in PVCs and resulted in suppression of ventricular tachycardia and fibrillation. Lown and Graboys (228) in their report on malignant ventricular arrhythmias (ventricular fibrillation or ventricular tachycardia with syncope) treated three patients with MVP out of 43 consecutive patients (7%) with such arrhythmias, and found that Norpace® (disopyramide phosphate) in a daily dose of 600 mg completely abolished all advanced grades of ventricular arrhythmias in one of their patients with MVP. In this 39-year-old woman who had numerous episodes of ventricular fibrillation, other antiarrhythmic drugs and overdrive pacing were without benefit. Twenty-nine months after institution of Norpace® therapy, the patient was leading a normal life and had not experienced any recurrence of her arrhythmia. However, another patient with MVP and refractory ventricular tachycardia due to ectopic pacemaker (134) died 4 months after institution of a high dose of disopyramide phosphate therapy. In Lown's patient the acetylstrophantidin tolerance test strikingly reduced PVCs. The efficacy of digitalis in the management of PVCs in this syndrome has not been thoroughly investigated.

The systematic approach to the management of malignant ventricular arrhythmias advocated by Lown and Graboys (228) deserves serious consideration and may become widely accepted in MVP associated with such arrhythmias. It is based on acute drug testing followed by drug usage over 48 to 72 hr with drug efficacy determined with use of ambulatory monitoring and exercise stress. These investigators use programmed trendscription for the "expeditious screening of drugs for efficacy as well as appropriate dose." They stress the fact that drug combinations should be tried and that abolition of all ectopic activity is not necessary for therapeutic success.

Should antiarrhythmic drugs, singly or in combination, fail to control malignant arrhythmias in this syndrome, consideration should be given to pacing. In such instances, a trial with a temporary pacemaker should be instituted before the placement of a permanent pacemaker. Ritchie et al. (301) have successfully used overdrive pacing to prevent arrhythmias in a 56-year-old man who had repeated attacks of ventricular fibrillation. Kremkau et al. (206) have successfully used permanent transvenous ventricular pacing in a 32-year-old woman with multifocal PVCs and bursts of ventricular tachycardia that were extremely difficult to control; propranolol therapy was maintained in conjunction with pacing. Mills et al. (253) have also successfully used pacing and three antidysrhythmic agents in a 26-year-old woman who had been successfully resuscitated from ventricular fibrillation; this combination "has resulted in a symptom-free period of 5 years." Likewise, we have found long term pacing effective in the management of arrhythmia in a 60-year-old woman with recurrent ventricular tachycardia and syncope refractory to various antiarrhythmic drugs. A syncopal episode during one of her numerous hospital admissions was probably due to ventricular fibrillation that converted with chest thump. Neither click nor murmur were heard. Pronounced prolapse of both leaflets was noted on left ventriculography and the coronary arteriogram was normal. The patient has had no recurrence of syncope during a 20-month follow-up period. EKG now shows an artificial pacemaker rhythm at 89 beats/min with no evidence of PVCs (Fig. 8.16).

Other workers [Guthrie and Edwards quoted in ref. 175 and Lown and Graboys (228)] have not had the same success with pacing.

Mitral valve replacement for prevention of life threatening arrhythmias was performed in five patients who had ventricular fibrillation (73,380) including a patient of Dr. Paul N. Yu (case not yet reported). A 40-year-old woman [Case 1 of Cobbs and King (73)] underwent mitral valve replacement after a "prolonged near fatal episode of ventricular fibrillation." PVCs disappeared almost completely for almost 3 months but then recurred, finally responding to a combination of propranolol and diphenylhydantoin; 24 months postoperatively the patient was leading a normal life and the standard and post exercise EKGs were virtually normal. A second patient reported by the same authors, a 59-year-old woman, underwent mitral valve replacement after several episodes of ventricular fibrillation recurring despite combined propranolol and diphenylhydantoin therapy; during an 18-month postoperative follow-up, "previously inverted T waves have normalized and arrhythmias have not re-

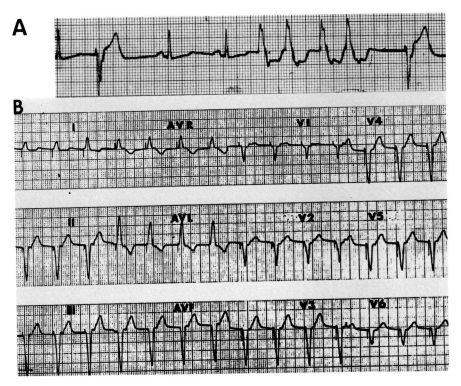

FIG. 8.16. *Case 247.* Effect of pacing on intractable ventricular arrhythmias and recurrent syncope in a 60-year-old woman with "silent" MVP and normal coronary arteriogram (see text). A. EKG prior to pacing—Multiform PVCs and salvo of four PVCs (see Fig. 8.11.A). B. Pacing at a rate of 88/min. Premature ventricular activity was abolished.

curred." In a third case, a 70-year-old woman with MVP and severe mitral regurgitation, multiple syncopal episodes due to ventricular fibrillation had occurred; mitral valve replacement was carried out but propranolol and diphenylhydantoin therapy had to be maintained because of recurrence of ventricular fibrillation when this drug regimen was discontinued. Eighteen months postoperatively arrhythmias have not recurred. No information has been published by Dr. Yu on his patient. The fifth patient to undergo mitral valve replacement (380) had recurrent ventricular fibrillation with severe mitral regurgitation; 5 years later ventricular fibrillation had not recurred but the patient had required continued antiarrhythmic therapy.

Mitral valve replacement should be considered only as a life saving measure in patients with recurrent episodes of ventricular tachycardia and fibrillation unresponsive to antiarrhythmic therapy and pacing. The antiarrhythmic protocol advocated by Lown and Graboys (228) should be implemented before embarking on this drastic method of treatment. The efficacy of mitral valve replacement in abolishing arrhythmias should be investigated by comparing the prevalence of arrhythmias prior to and after surgery in patients requiring mitral valve replacement for mitral valve prolapse and severe mitral insufficiency.

Atrial arrhythmias in this syndrome should be managed with digitalis, quinidine, propranolol, and so forth. Identification of preexcitation as the underlying mechanism of the arrhythmia in some of these patients would require the mode of therapy and the precautions dictated by this disorder (133). Drugs such as digitalis and propranolol may be dangerous in the presence of antegrade conduction over an atrioventricular bypass tract (183). Should atrial fibrillation or flutter develop in these patients, digitalis may facilitate conduction over the bypass tract and lead to ventricular fibrillation.

There is a paucity of information on the management of bradyarrhythmias in MVP. Propranolol therapy is contraindicated if significant bradyarrhythmias of sinoatrial or atrioventricular nodes origin are identified. Five patients (149,217,234) have required permanent pacing for syncope associated with severe sinus bradycardia or complete AV block.

INDICATIONS FOR ANTIARRHYTHMIC THERAPY IN MVP

Arrhythmias, particularly PVCs, are common in MVP and yet sudden death is a rare occurrence. These contrasting findings would not favor aggressive management of all the arrhythmias encountered in this syndrome. In general, the prognostic significance of arrhythmias, particularly PVCs, depends on the underlying cardiac disorder: PVCs are usually of no consequence in the absence of heart disease, but carry serious connotations in coronary artery disease and particularly in acute myocardial infarction. At this time, it is impossible to determine, from the available evidence, in which prognostic category the PVCs in MVP fall. This should not be surprising given the controversy still surrounding PVCs in coronary artery disease, their significance, prognostic implications, identification as marker of sudden death, and the efficacy of their suppression in the prevention of sudden death. The extensive investigations carried out in coronary artery disease have not yet solved this problem. Research into the significance of PVCs in MVP will be facilitated by the prevalence of this syndrome and of the associated arrhythmias but it will be hampered by the rare occurrence of life threatening arrhythmias and sudden death to be prevented. The side effects of most antiarrhythmic agents and the lack of an ideal antiarrhythmic drug further complicate any aggressive therapeutic approach to the arrhythmias in MVP.

It remains to be determined if multiform repetitive or early PVCs have ominous significance and require the same aggressive management that is advocated when they are associated with coronary artery disease. The frequency of PVCs (more than 20–30 per hour) in this syndrome (228,384,386) may be associated with a high incidence of ventricular tachycardia and may warrant antiarrhythmic therapy.

In summary, whether or not complex and frequent PVCs in MVP "have the same ominous prognosis as for patients with coronary artery disease will need to be determined by prospective long term follow-up studies involving a large number of patients" (384). This determination would allow us to better define the indications for antiarrhythmic treatment in this syndrome. Until such studies are available, antiarrhythmic therapy is recommended in the following patients:

1. Patients with symptomatic and distressing arrhythmias, including frequent palpitations, dizziness, and particularly syncope (if they are shown to be associated with arrhythmia by ambulatory monitoring).

2. Patients with frequent PVCs (more than 30 per hour) particularly if they are multiform and if they abut or interrupt the T waves. This recommendation is based on the association of ventricular tachycardia with preceding frequent PVCs and extrapolation of data in coronary artery disease to MVP. Its rationale is, therefore, open to controversy.

3. Patients who have sustained ventricular tachycardia and fibrillation.

Antiarrhythmic therapy is not warranted in the great majority of patients with MVP because their symptoms are either mild or unrelated to arrhythmia, and their arrhythmia, when present, consists mostly of benign PVCs of slight to moderate frequency. Since most people with MVP are young or middle-aged adults, the initiation of antiarrhythmic therapy might imply exposure to various drugs for lengthy periods. As stated by Swartz et al. (355): "the physician must weigh the risks of antiarrhythmic therapy against the risk of morbidity without therapy in each individual patient. No generalization can, therefore, be made."

Chapter 9

Echocardiographic Features

Echocardiography, a widely used noninvasive technique, has joined auscultation and angiography as the third diagnostic marker in MVP. It is particularly useful in the diagnosis of the "silent" form of this syndrome and in the demonstration of prolapse when the click is early or evanescent, or when isolated late systolic or pansystolic murmurs are heard. In the diagnosis of idiopathic MVP associated with coronary artery disease, echocardiography is more helpful than left ventriculography, which yields nonspecific findings shared by papillary muscle dysfunction and idiopathic MVP. The sensitivity, specificity, and predictive value of echocardiography have not been established and considerable controversy continues to surround the echocardiographic criteria of MVP.

Shah and Gramiak (331), Dillon et al. (109) and Kerber et al. (191) were the first investigators to describe the echocardiographic findings in MVP and to stress the usefulness of M mode echocardiography in the diagnosis of this syndrome. Shah and Gramiak (331) deserve full credit for having outlined, as early as in 1970, the two main echocardiographic features of MVP (i.e., posterior midsystolic dipping of the leaflet or a "hammock like" generalized posterior displacement). Since publication of these papers in 1970 and 1971, there has been an information explosion on the subject of echocardiographic recognition of MVP (39,43,44,45,61,63,64,65, 74,99,100,101,123,125,138,141,145,146,166,233,236,238,241,242,254,255, 262,266,280,282,283,284,289,314,315,316,331,342,372,373,378,381) yet the "ultrasound diagnosis of the mitral valve prolapse syndrome continues to be one of the principal unresolved areas in echocardiography today" (101).

NORMAL MOVEMENT OF THE MITRAL VALVE ON M MODE ECHOCARDIOGRAM (FIGS. 9.1 AND 9.2)

With the onset of ventricular contraction the two mitral leaflets come into apposition (point C). During systole, the anterior and posterior leaflets remain close together and move anteriorly, reflecting the anterior movement of the mitral ring as the left ventricle empties (CD segment). This normal anterior movement of both leaflets is disturbed by the presence of prolapse. At the beginning of diastole the two leaflets separate, the anterior leaflet moving to point E. After E the anterior leaflet moves posteriorly (E–F

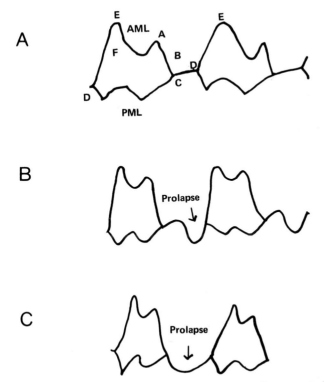

FIG. 9.1. Diagram of normal mitral valve echocardiogram (A), of late systolic (B) and holosystolic prolapse (C). AML, Anterior mitral leaflet; PML, posterior mitral leaflet.

slope), and remains in a semiclosed position until the atrial contraction re-opens it and it moves anteriorly to point A. With the beginning of ventricular contraction the leaflet moves posteriorly to point C, where it meets the posterior leaflet. The latter leaflet moves in the opposite fashion during diastole. It is not unusual to record multiple echoes from the mitral valve during systole but they rarely number more than three and characteristically they manifest parallel motion (101).

ECHOCARDIOGRAPHIC FINDINGS IN MVP

Posterior buckling of the mitral leaflets in midsystole is accepted by most workers as the diagnostic hallmark of the MVP syndrome (Figs 9.3 to 9.5). This finding was first described by Dillon et al. (109) and Kerber et al. (191) in their pioneering studies and was reported as "quite specific" (109) and "characteristic" (191). The abrupt posterior motion results in a

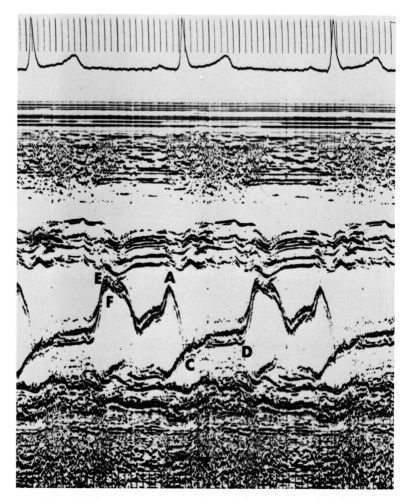

FIG. 9.2. Normal mitral echogram. Note normal anterior movement of both mitral leaflets during systole (CD). (See text).

configuration that resembles a question mark turned approximately 90° clockwise (282). Multiple echoes are frequently seen, and accentuation of the degree of buckling in each succeeding posterior echo is characteristically noted. Approximately one-half of patients with abrupt midsystolic buckling exhibit a straight or anterior motion in early systole prior to the posterior dipping; the other half manifest posterior movement of the leaflet from the onset of systole with a superimposed backward buckling in midsystole (101). The midsystolic buckling is not noted in patients with MVP and ruptured chordae who exhibit pansystolic "hammocking."

Pansystolic bowing or hammocking was first noted by Shah and associates

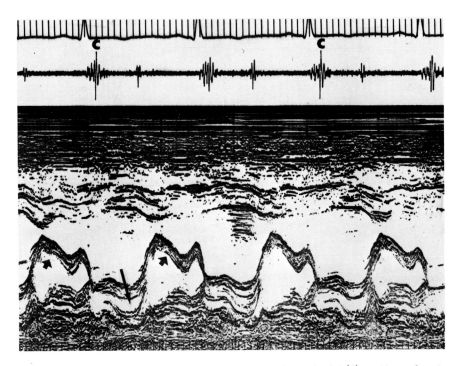

FIG. 9.3. *Case 334.* Echocardiogram in a young woman with early systolic click (C) provides confirmation of MVP. Marked midsystolic buckling *(lower arrow)* and multiple systolic echoes are seen. Note thick cusps and shaggy echoes behind anterior leaflet in the absence of endocarditis *(upper arrows).*

(331) and subsequently by Popp and colleagues (282) and DeMaria and associates (91,101) (Figs. 9.6A, 9.6B, 9.7 and 9.8). In their most recent series, DeMaria et al. (101) reported that 66% of their patients with auscultatory findings of MVP manifested midsystolic buckling whereas 34% exhibited pansystolic hammocking. However, in an earlier series of 33 patients with MVP documented by biplane left ventricular angiography the same authors had reported that pansystolic bowing was the most frequent echocardiographic abnormality in this syndrome. Characteristically, the bowing motion begins early in systole at the C point and reaches its nadir in the middle of systole (U shaped deformity). Patients with dilated cardiomyopathy may show a flat systolic segment on the echocardiogram which deviates less than 2 mm from a line connecting the C and D points (280). This echo appearance can be distinguished from MVP by the occurrence of insignificant posterior motion of the leaflets (less than 2 mm) and has been attributed to "so little change in volume during systole that the anterior migration of the mitral valve may be nearly imperceptible" (282).

In addition to midsystolic buckling and pansystolic bowing, a marked posterior motion of the leaflet echo close to the left atrial wall and visible

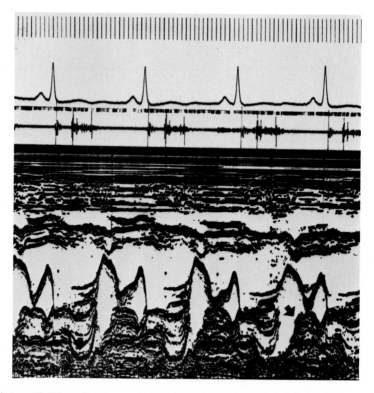

FIG. 9.4. *Case 40.* Echocardiogram in a 28-year-old woman with multiple clicks and late systolic murmur (Phonocardiogram beneath EKG). Marked midsystolic buckling of both leaflets (*left arrow*): onset of buckling coincides with the first and loudest click. Note heavy diastolic echoes behind posterior leaflet (*right arrow*).

more than 50% of systole has been found to correlate well with other evidence of MVP (99,101,233). This movement, termed "localized mitral collapse" (99) was noted in the sectors traversing the mitral leaflets and left atrium and was described as "a precipitous plunging or backward collapse of the anterior leaflet to meet the posterior leaflet against the left atrial wall" (99). A similar echocardiographic finding can be noted on scanning from the heart toward the aorta: fragments of the prolapsed leaflets can then be seen in the left atrium even though the sector of the aortic leaflets is seen (101).

The midsystolic buckling is so characteristic of MVP and correlates so well with the auscultatory and angiographic findings that most workers in this field would accept it as diagnostic of this syndrome in the absence of auscultatory or typical angiographic findings. Conversely, the pansystolic bowing or hammocking remains a controversial finding as to significance and diagnostic value (123). In some patients with MVP proven by auscultation or angiography, pansystolic hammocking may alternate with midsystolic

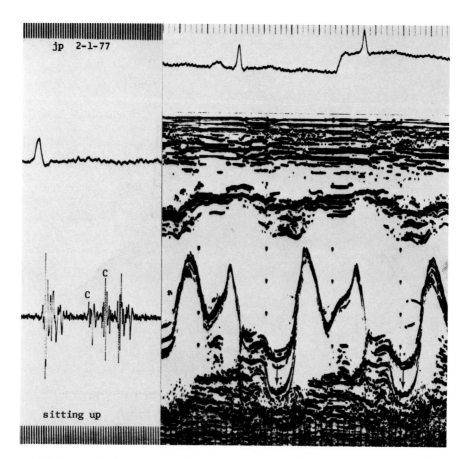

FIG. 9.5. *Case 311.* Echocardiogram and phonocardiogram in a 22-year-old woman. Multiple systolic clicks (C) are seen. Marked midsystolic buckling (arrow) is evident. Note increased excursion of the anterior mitral leaflet.

buckling during the same study depending on the transducer position. Yet in a definite proportion of patients with MVP, pansystolic bowing may be the "solitary ultrasound manifestation" (101) despite diligent echocardiographic scanning from multiple transducer positions.

The specificity of the pansystolic hammocking can be strengthened by requiring a pronounced degree of bowing, and by rigid definition of the timing of the bowing movement. With regard to the depth of hammocking, Markiewicz and associates (233) described a 2 mm deviation from a line connecting the C and D points of the mitral valve echogram as satisfying their criteria for MVP. I believe that this minimal degree of bowing results in loss of specificity and in a higher percentage of false positive echocardiographic diagnosis. Others (36) tightened their criteria and required a posterior displacement of 5 mm or greater. Requiring 5 mm posterior displacement

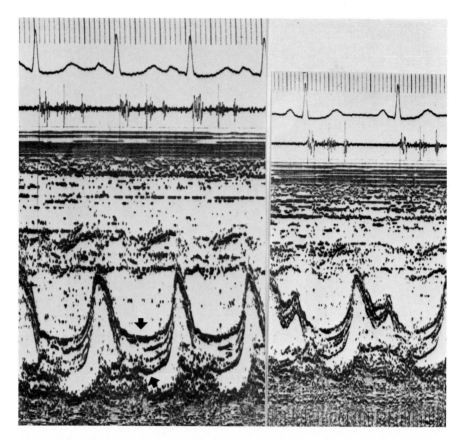

FIG. 9.6A. *Case 336. Echocardiogram in a 47-year-old woman with multiple clicks (phono beneath EKG); marked hammocking (arrow) is evident.*

increases the specificity of this echocardiographic finding but would impair its sensitivity. A 3 mm posterior displacement would seem, in my opinion, to be a more reasonable criterion that would yield an acceptable sensitivity and specificity. The specificity of "hammocking" is enhanced by requiring a continuous smooth movement that begins at the onset of systole with its nadir occurring at midsystole (101). A slight early movement just following the C point with subsequent straight gradual anterior motion of the mitral valve leaflet does not correlate with other evidence of MVP (101) (Fig. 9.9). A minimal late systolic dipping of the mitral leaflets of less than 2 mm when measured from the C point is probably a nonspecific finding and has not been found to correlate with the auscultatory findings (233) (Fig. 9.10).

More extensive studies of specificity and sensitivity are needed but they will suffer from the lack of an adequate "gold standard" for the diagnosis of MVP. The angiographic criteria themselves suffer from the same controversy

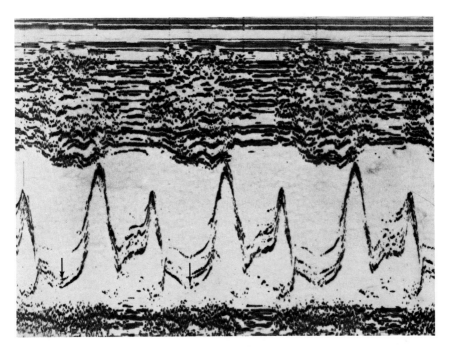

FIG. 9.6B. *Case 176.* Marked pansystolic sagging (arrow) in a 50-year-old patient with a midsystolic click. Note multiple systolic echoes and wide diastolic excursion of the anterior leaflet.

surrounding the echocardiographic criteria and require further refinement and quantitation. The auscultatory criteria (i.e., the detection of a nonejection click) have the advantages of long and extensive experience but their specificity for MVP is based primarily on auscultatory–pathological correlation in only 26 patients reported in the literature (see Chaps. 3 and 4). I believe, therefore, that the establishment of echocardiographic criteria should be based on correlation with auscultatory findings (i.e., clicks), and on confirmatory angiograms when available. DeMaria et al. (101) reported on such correlation and their studies should be expanded.

With the introduction of new diagnostic techniques, physicians tend to be too demanding of the new diagnostic tool, overlooking the lack of specificity and sensitivity of other useful techniques in their armamentarium. Suffice to mention the controversy that still surrounds standard and exercise electrocardiography. Symmetrically and deeply inverted T waves are generally accepted as indicative of ischemia, but we have learned to interpret more shallow and less symmetrical T waves as nonspecific, nondiagnostic, and requiring clinical correlations. We should transpose this electrocardiographic jargon to the description of echocardiographic findings and stop insisting on the black and white concept while overlooking the gray zone that engulfs each diagnostic technique.

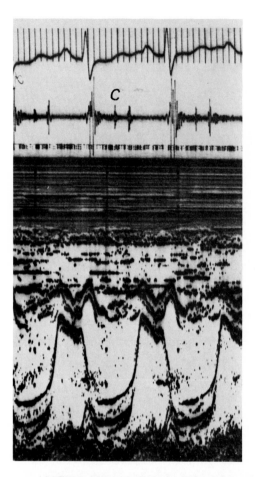

FIG. 9.7. Case 333. Echocardiogram in a young woman with a mid to late systolic click (c). Marked hammocking is evident, with no temporal correlation between click and either onset of sagging, or maximal posterior excursion of leaflet.

ANCILLARY ECHOCARDIOGRAPHIC FEATURES OF MVP

Various ancillary echocardiographic findings have been described as supporting the diagnosis of MVP. Increased amplitude of excursion of the anterior leaflet of 25 mm or greater is frequently encountered in MVP (100,101,123) and results in the anterior leaflet abutting upon the interventricular septum in early diastole. Multiple systolic leaflets echoes, usually greater than three, are frequently encountered and correspond probably to the redundancy and multiscalloped appearance of the leaflets (101,282). Occasionally, the mitral leaflets may appear thickened (101).

TECHNICAL ASPECTS OF ECHOCARDIOGRAPHIC DIAGNOSIS OF MVP

Correct placement of the transducer is a prerequisite for accurate echocardiographic diagnosis of MVP (44,101,233,238). Only the "perpendicu-

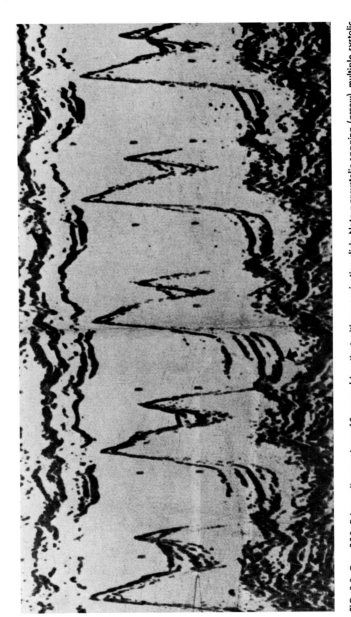

FIG. 9.8. Case 288. Echocardiogram in an 18-year-old patient with a nonejection click. Note pansystolic sagging (arrow), multiple systolic echoes, and marked increase in the diastolic excursion of the anterior leaflet.

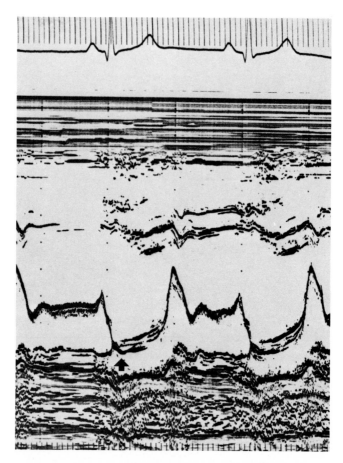

FIG. 9.9. Echocardiogram in a 19-year-old patient with aortic insufficiency. Note early systolic dipping with subsequent normal anterior movement of the mitral leaflet (*arrow*). This tracing is not diagnostic of MVP (101), because in MVP, the nadir of the hammocking occurs in midsystole.

lar" transducer position should be used when analyzing echocardiograms for the presence of MVP. In this position, the transducer is either perpendicular to the chest in the sagittal plane or pointing slightly cephalad. With the transducer high on the chest and pointing caudally when both mitral leaflets and atrium are recorded, holosystolic posterior motion of the mitral leaflets is noted in a high percentage of normal subjects, yielding, therefore, a false positive diagnosis of MVP. In this position, the D point is posterior to the C point. Conversely, with the transducer pointing cephalad a posterior displacement of the posterior leaflet is never seen and an anterior systolic deviation is frequently noted masking the typical findings of MVP (Fig. 9.11). In this position, the D point is anterior to the C point. The third intercostal space appears to be the point of choice in most patients provided that an

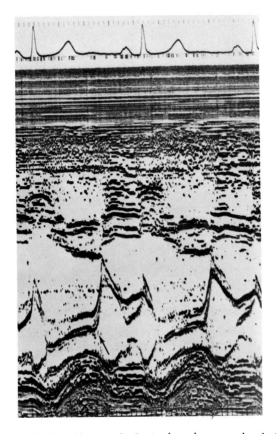

FIG. 9.10. Minimal late systolic dipping (arrow)—a normal variant.

adequate study can be obtained with the transducer in perpendicular position (233). The effect of transducer placement can be explained by the downward and anterior movement of the base of the heart including the mitral valve ring and the mitral leaflets during systole (233). With the ultrasonic beam coming from a high interspace and pointing caudally, the mitral ring and leaflets move perpendicular to the beam or even away from the transducer so the echocardiogram may register a posterior displacement of the mitral leaflets. An anterior motion of the mitral leaflets can be registered with the transducer located in a low interspace pointing cephalad; in this position, MVP will rarely be recorded.

For optimal demonstration of MVP, both mitral leaflets should be recorded in front of the left atrium (101,233,282). As pointed out by Popp et al. (282) echoes from both mitral leaflets in MVP can be recorded clearly with the sound beam directed up through the valve area and into the

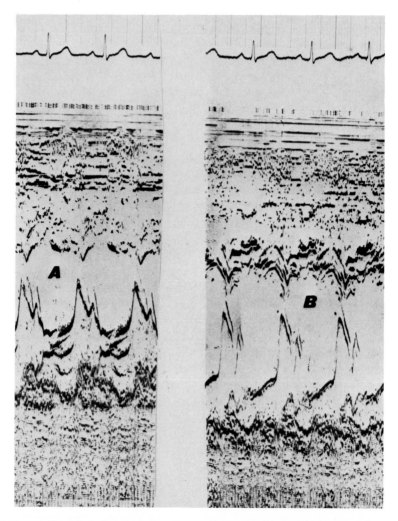

FIG. 9.11. Case 338. Effect of transducer position on echocardiographic manifestation of MVP. A. Transducer in the "perpendicular" position. Midsystolic buckling is noted. B. Transducer in a lower interspace pointing cephalad; the echocardiographic evidence of MVP is masked. Note that the D point is anterior to the C point.

left atrium unlike other groups of patients in whom simultaneous recording of the posterior leaflet and the left atrium is unusual. The same authors stress the difficulty in recognizing the posterior systolic motion of the mitral valve in MVP on echocardiogram displaying simultaneously the left ventricular posterior wall due to the normal anterior systolic motion of this wall. They suggest that the transducer be placed lower than the usual position on the chest wall so that "the sound beam will pass up through the mitral valve structures and into the left atrium." However, it should be noted that in this low position and with the transducer pointing cephalad, the echocardio-graphic feature of MVP may be obstructed. Maximal prolapse is frequently seen at the junction of the left atrium and left ventricle (123) and in some patients, typical findings of MVP are only noted on an M mode scan from the left ventricle to the aorta (123).

The maximum prolapsing echo is frequently less intense that the other echoes, is the most posterior, and can be missed if the gain is too low (123) (Fig. 6.13). Isolated prolapse of the posterior leaflet is not uncommon, and therefore, echocardiographic visualization of this leaflet is required before MVP can be ruled out.

SIGNIFICANCE OF SYSTOLIC SEPARATION OF ANTERIOR AND POSTERIOR LEAFLETS

Dillon et al. (109) reported an association between mitral insufficiency and systolic separation of the two mitral leaflets on echocardiography, and felt that this separation was indicative of mitral regurgitation in patients with MVP. Other workers (145,282) were unable to confirm this finding. Apparent separation of anterior and posterior leaflet echoes may be recorded without auscultatory or angiographic findings of mitral regurgitation, and therefore does not correlate with the presence of mitral regurgitation. In most cases, the apparent separation of the leaflets results from the presence of multiple parallel echoes, a frequent finding in MVP (282).

ECHOCARDIOGRAPHIC IDENTIFICATION OF THE PROLAPSED LEAFLET

Multiple echoes originating from both leaflets in MVP make identification of the prolapsed leaflets difficult (99,145). Despite the original emphasis on the posterior leaflet as the site of prolapse, recent echocardiographic studies stressed the frequency of prolapse of both leaflets (74,99,282). DeMaria et al. (99) were able to identify abnormal posterior motion of both leaflets in 23 of their 27 patients with MVP (85%). Likewise, Cohen et al. (74) stressed the common occurrence of double mitral leaflet prolapse that was noted in 19 of their 35 patients (54%). They felt that this figure was likely to be an underestimate since echocardiographic studies that did not really define both leaflets were considered to be representative of single leaflet prolapse. In Chap. 3, I stressed the frequency of involvement of both leaflets in MVP. Yet the frequency of both leaflets prolapsing on echocardiography is substantially greater than the occurrence of morphological abnormalities of both mitral leaflets (99). This discrepancy can be attributed to the de-pendence of each leaflet upon the other leaflet with which it coapts for proper function, and perhaps to chordal involvement in the disease process since the chordae originating from each papillary muscle insert into both mitral cusps.

RELATIVE FREQUENCY OF DETECTION OF MVP IN ECHOCARDIOGRAPHIC LABORATORIES

The frequency of detection of MVP in an echocardiographic laboratory depends on the diagnostic criteria employed. If minimal hammocking is accepted as diagnostic of MVP, then a high percentage of the cases studied will be labeled as MVP. The reported frequency of MVP diagnosis varies from 6% in one laboratory (101), to 10% in another laboratory (74), and to as high as 12% in a third (146). These studies refer to a select group of patients who are evaluated for symptoms and auscultatory abnormalities. The prevalence of MVP in the general population was discussed in Chap. 2.

SENSITIVITY OF M MODE ECHOCARDIOGRAPHY IN MVP

I have already reviewed available data on the specificity of the echocardiographic findings in MVP. The sensitivity of M mode echocardiography suffers from the inherent deficiency of this technique which aims a single beam at the mitral valve and may not, therefore, depict localized prolapse that may involve a single scallop of the posterior leaflet (Figs. 9.12 and 9.13). Wigle et al. (380) reported observations indicating that M mode echocardiography probably strikes the middle scallop of the posterior leaflet as well as the anterior leaflet; thus prolapse of the posteromedial and of the anterolateral scallops of the posterior leaflet could be missed. Despite this shortcoming, M mode echocardiography has been found to be a highly sensitive diagnostic technique in MVP. For instance, DeMaria et al. (101) were able to record "an echocardiographic abnormality in 90% of the patients with the auscultatory findings of midsystolic click and/or late systolic murmur"; the echocardiographic abnormality in some of these patients was a pansystolic hammocking that, unfortunately, suffers from a lack of specificity. Markiewicz et al. (233) reported a similarly high sensitivity of 82% in their studies of 17 females with midsystolic click, late systolic murmur, with 35% of these 17 patients showing the specific echocardiographic pattern of midsystolic buckling, 47% the less specific pansystolic sagging of 2 mm or more, and the remainder other variants. Malcolm et al. (231) reported a 75% sensitivity. My experience would confirm the high sensitivity of echocardiography in MVP (80%); however, about 50% of my patients were found to have pansystolic sagging, the less specific of the 2 echocardiographic criteria.

Using angiographic criteria, other workers (39,314) reported a lower sensitivity for echocardiography in MVP. Boughner et al. (39) studied 43 patients with angiographically proven MVP and found that echocardiography

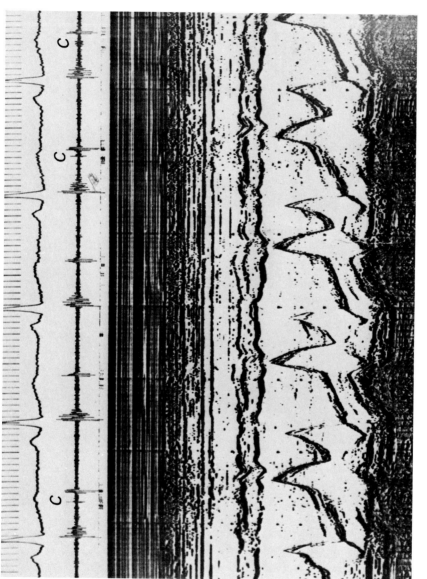

FIG. 9.12. Case 332. Normal echocardiogram despite the presence of an intermittent late systolic click (arrows).

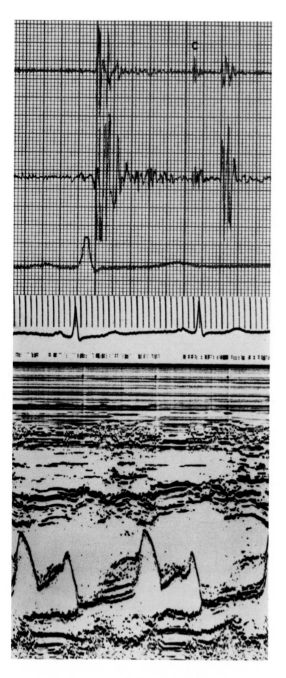

FIG. 9.13. Case 337. Normal echo-cardiogram in a young woman with a mid to late systolic click (C).

showed "definite" MVP (midsystolic buckling in 10 (24%) and "probable" MVP (hammocking) in 13 (30%), giving a total sensitivity of 54%. In their experience, echocardiography was least reliable when only the postero-medial commissural scallop was involved. Unfortunately, these authors did not report on the auscultatory findings in their patients and on the frequency of coronary artery disease that is commonly associated with angiographic MVP but with negative echocardiography (echocardiographic–angiographic discordance). Likewise, Ruwitch et al. (314) reported on the insensitivity of echocardiography in detecting MVP in older patients with chest pain. In 11 patients with a mean age of 47 years with moderate to severe MVP confirmed angiographically and with normal coronary arteriogram, echocardiography revealed MVP in only one case, was probably negative in two, and was clearly negative in eight. Since an early systolic click was detected in only three patients and a mid or late systolic murmur or both in only five, most of these patients, therefore, did not manifest the midsystolic click, the auscultatory hallmark of MVP, and this negative finding detracts from the value of this study. The authors point out that their patients were relatively older, more predominantly male, and that in most of them it was technically difficult to record the echocardiogram because of large anteroposterior chest dimension, and because these patients offered "a limited number of transducer positions from which the mitral valve could be seen well enough to "search" for subtle evidence of prolapse."

From the above studies, I would conclude that further work is needed for evaluation of the sensitivity of echocardiography in MVP. There is a discrepancy between results of studies based on auscultatory versus angiographic evidence of MVP. Echocardiography was found less sensitive in the angiographic studies raising the often asked question: does angiography provide the "gold standard" for the diagnosis of MVP? The subject will be discussed in Chap. 12. Evaluation of the sensitivity of echocardiography should probably be based on the finding of a nonejection click in the group being studied. Angiographic demonstration of MVP in this group when available would add further confirmation. Pure angiographic criteria should be used only when they are definite and in the absence of coronary artery disease.

Negative echocardiography in MVP may be due to several factors. The most important is the quality of the tracing and the impossibility of obtaining an adequate study or of visualizing the posterior leaflet in all patients. Another factor is the position of the transducer with masking of MVP if the transducer is located too low on the chest and points cephalad. I have already mentioned a third factor (the single beam or "icepick view"), which does not visualize each scallop of the redundant leaflet, as an inherent limitation in the sensitivity of echocardiography in MVP. Moreover, recent data from two-dimensional echocardiography indicates that a major component of prolapse occurs in a cephalad rather than a true posterior direction, but only abnormal posterior motion is demonstrated by M mode echocardiography.

INDICATIONS FOR ECHOCARDIOGRAPHY: DIAGNOSTIC IMPLICATIONS

In the presence of a nonejection click confirmed by phonocardiography, echocardiography is not required to establish the diagnosis of MVP. The click is generally accepted as the diagnostic hallmark of idiopathic MVP and pathological corroboration of its diagnostic significance, albeit in only 26 cases, is most impressive. The specificity of the click as a diagnostic marker of idiopathic MVP has been confirmed by echocardiography, which has been found positive in 80 to 90% of patients with nonejection clicks and by angiography, which I found diagnostic of MVP in each of the 35 patients with nonejection clicks that I studied. Therefore, the demonstration of a positive echocardiogram when a click is noted is redundant and does not add helpful information. However, if the click is early or the murmur is pansystolic or late systolic without associated click, echocardiographic or angiographic confirmation is essential for the diagnosis of MVP. Echocardiography as a noninvasive technique would constitute the simplest, cheapest, and safest diagnostic method in these instances. Moreover, since the sensitivity of echocardiography in MVP is at the most in the 80% range, a negative echocardiogram in the presence of a click does not rule out MVP. To quote Dr. James A. Ronan, Jr.: "An echocardiogram that does not show mitral valve prolapse does not exclude it. In fact, it is not uncommon for the subject with the systolic click without a murmur to have a negative echocardiogram. So much depends on the skill of the echocardiographer and the correct placement of the beam exactly on the affected area. Small areas of mitral valve prolapse can be easily missed. The auscultatory evidence of the syndrome is no less valuable than the echocardiographic evidence. Believe your ears!" (264). I would add: but get phonocardiographic confirmation because the click may be evanescent and others may not believe your ears.

When the diagnosis of MVP is made on the basis of left ventriculography alone, echocardiography provides further confirmation of MVP particularly if the angiogram is not clearly diagnostic. Controversies continue to surround the angiographic diagnostic criteria for MVP especially when they are borderline and when only one scallop of the posterior leaflet is involved. Because of this, a positive echocardiogram would add valuable diagnostic information. In the absence of a click, echocardiography provides the only noninvasive means of diagnosing "silent" MVP. Strict echocardiography criteria should be adhered to, relying primarily on midsystolic buckling. To be of predictive value pansystolic sagging should be obvious exceeding 3 mm and with its nadir in midsystole. I concur with DeMaria and Mason's statement: "If the echogram is the solitary abnormality and is not of the midsystolic buckling variety, the patients are advised that they have an atypical cardiac finding of uncertain significance" (100). The degree of pansystolic sagging, the associated ancillary abnormalities (i.e., increased diastolic excursion of the anterior leaflet and multiple systolic echoes) add confirmatory evidence to the suspicion of MVP in such cases. Clinical correlation is also most helpful. The occurrence of pansystolic sagging is consistent with MVP when it is encountered in a young woman with chest deformity, chest pain, palpitations, arrhythmia, T wave changes in the inferior leads, and so forth.

Echocardiography is indicated in searching for MVP in patients with atypical chest pain, arrhythmias, and abnormal EKG, particularly if the inferior leads are involved. Transient ischemic attacks in a young subject may become an indication for echocardiography in order to search for underlying MVP (21).

CORRELATIONS OF ECHOCARDIOGRAPHY
WITH VARIOUS AUSCULTATORY FINDINGS

Although Shah and Gramiak (331) reported a correlation between echocardiographic and phonocardiographic finding (i.e., association of abrupt displacement in midsystole with midsystolic click and late systolic murmur, and of "hammocking" with holosystolic murmur), most investigators found no correlation between the echocardiographic type of MVP and the auscultatory findings (74,99,101,282) (Fig. 9.7). In one series (99), for instance, of 14 patients with pansystolic sagging on echocardiography pansystolic murmurs were noted in only two patients, midsystolic click and/or late systolic murmur in five, multiple clicks with late systolic murmur in two, early click in four, and no auscultatory abnormality in one patient. In this same series, there was a better correlation between midsystolic prolapse and the midsystolic click and/or late systolic murmur that were recorded in 10 of the 12 patients with these echocardiographic features. Cohen (74) also reported no apparent correlation between the echocardiographic and phonocardiographic finding: pansystolic murmurs were present in three patients with midsystolic prolapse, and midsystolic click and late systolic murmur in two patients with pansystolic prolapse.

It is not infrequent to note midsystolic and pansystolic prolapse with different transducer positions in the same echocardiographic tracing (101) in patients with either click, late systolic, or pansystolic murmurs. The mitral valve is a complex bileaflet, multiscalloped, parachute-like structure, and the single echo beam is unable to visualize all portions of the valve simultaneously (383) to provide meaningful echocardiographic–phonocardiographic correlations. Discrepancies between auscultatory abnormalities and the single beam echocardiogram "may reflect varied patterns of prolapse in different portions of the mitral leaflets, an occurrence demonstrated by multiple crystal echocardiography" (108,316).

Although no correlation has been reported between the type of echocardiographic MVP and the auscultatory findings, a temporal relationship has been noted between the phonocardiographic and echocardiographic events in the same patient. Winkle et al. (383), using simultaneous echocardiographic–phonocardiographic recordings at rest and during amyl nitrite administration, have reported that the initial vibrations of the auscultatory phenomena occur after the onset of echocardiographic prolapse but prior to maximal echocardiographic prolapse. The peak intensity of the clicks usually coincides with the point of maximal prolapse. In this same study, and in an earlier study by Dillon et al. (109), all patients with late systolic prolapse on echocardiography had the onset of MVP occurring earlier in systole during amyl nitrite administration and "this earlier prolapse corresponded to the earlier occurrence of the onset of auscultatory phenomena" (383). However, with amyl nitrite inhalation, only three of the 17 patients with late systolic prolapse developed holosystolic prolapse while the remaining 14 retained the late systolic prolapse. Paradoxically, propranolol, which results in delayed occurrence of the click (84), has no effect on either the echocardiographic patterns or the timing of MVP, despite a statistically significant increase in left ventricular volume (381).

EFFECT OF PREMATURE BEATS ON ECHOCARDIOGRAPHIC PATTERN OF MVP

A prolapse pattern on echocardiography was reported by one group (64) in 20 out of 50 patients with PVCs. The authors found normal mitral valve motion in 11 patients with supraventricular extrasystoles and felt that a small ventricular volume alone is not sufficient to produce valve prolapse. The echocardiographic tracing published by these authors to illustrate their findings showed, in my opinion, minimal early posterior systolic motion that does not meet the echocardiographic criteria for the diagnosis of MVP. An echocardiogram diagnostic of MVP with midsystolic buckling occurring during PVCs, in a patient without evidence of MVP on clinical examination, was published by another group (101) who stated, however, that "in their experience prolapse is induced by PVCs in only a small percentage of patients and that characteristically it consists of a posterior motion of minor amplitude." In my experience, PVCs in normal subjects are associated with minimal nondiagnostic early posterior systolic motion, but in patients with MVP they result in accentuation of the echocardiographic prolapse pattern. In some patients with midsystolic buckling, hammocking is noted during the PVCs (282).

PSEUDO PROLAPSE OF THE MITRAL VALVE IN PERICARDIAL EFFUSION AND IN MITRAL STENOSIS

False positive patterns of MVP on the echocardiogram, including midsystolic buckling of the mitral leaflets, have been observed in the presence of pericardial effusion (266,372). Normal mitral motion was noted after removal of the pericardial fluid. This pseudo prolapse results, probably, from the swinging motion of the heart in the pericardial fluid. A predominant posterior swing during systole gives rise to a prolapse pattern whereas a predominant anterior swing would be associated with a SAM suggestive of idiopathic hypertrophic subaortic stenosis (IHSS). The diagnosis of MVP or IHSS should therefore not be made in the presence of pericardial effusion.

In patients with mitral stenosis, pansystolic hammocking, and, more rarely, mid to late systolic dipping have been described by Nichol et al. (262) who ascribed them "to distortion of leaflet closure induced by the effect of mitral stenosis on the valve apparatus." In view of this finding, echocardiography is not a specific means to identify MVP in patients with mitral stenosis and the diagnosis of this combination should rely on auscultatory, angiographic, and pathological findings (375,380).

MISCELLANEOUS ECHOCARDIOGRAPHIC FINDINGS IN MVP

Low amplitude systolic humps can be observed and are somewhat reminiscent of those seen in IHSS (39,145,280). On two-dimensional echocardiography, the systolic anterior motion of the mitral valve in MVP was felt to be due to systolic anterior motion of chordae tendineae (289) or to superimposition of echoes derived from the anterior mitral annulus upon echoes from the posterosuperiorly prolapsed leaflets (315).

Heavy diastolic echoes behind the posterior mitral leaflet can be seen (123) particularly in patients with "floppy" mitral valve and originate, probably, from a vertically oriented thickened and redundant posterior leaflet (Fig. 9.14).

Early diastolic paradoxical anterior motion of the posterior leaflet was described in three patients with MVP with intact chordae tendineae (123, 255), and was felt not to be a reliable sign of ruptured chordae. I have observed this anterior motion, lasting throughout diastole, in five patients, with floppy mitral valve, intact chordae, and severe mitral regurgitation who required mitral valve replacement (Figs. 9.14 and 9.15). It is possible that the elongated chordae tendineae in "floppy" mitral valve provide little support to the posterior leaflet and cause the paradoxical anterior motion usually associated with ruptured chordae tendineae. In severe MVP or in ruptured chordae, the posterior leaflet or part of it move probably into the left atrium during systole (255), and in early diastole, it moves anteriorly and inferiorly in the direction of the left ventricle. This diastolic anterior movement, when associated with decreased E–F slope of the anterior leaflet in a few patients with MVP, severe mitral insufficiency, heart failure, and decreased left ventricular compliance, may mimic the findings in mitral stenosis. Because of these echocardiographic findings, mitral stenosis that may coexist with MVP (375) should be ruled out clinically, hemodynami-

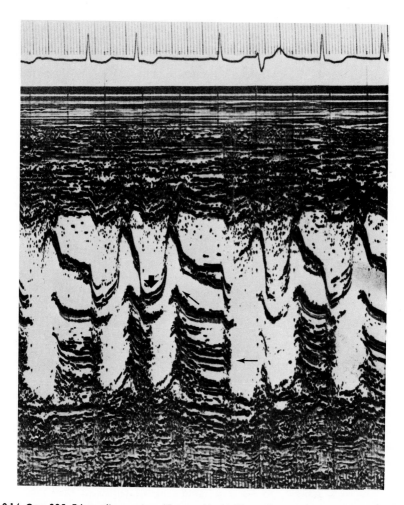

FIG. 9.14. *Case 335.* Echocardiogram in a 65-year-old with "floppy" mitral valve and severe mitral in-sufficiency, both confirmed at surgery. Chordae were intact. Note hammocking (*vertical arrow*), parodoxical anterior movement of the posterior leaflet in diastole (*oblique arrow*), and heavy echoes behind posterior leaflet (*horizontal arrow*). Atrial fibrillation is seen.

cally, or angiographically. According to Morcerf et al. (255) the diastolic anterior motion of the posterior leaflet in severe MVP can be differentiated from the movement in mitral stenosis by its faster velocity, which is even faster than the D–E slope of the anterior leaflet.

Thick, shaggy echoes similar to those generated by vegetations in infective endocarditis have been described in patients with MVP in the absence of clinical evidence of endocarditis (61,373) (Figs. 9.3 and 14.8). They limit the reliability of the echocardiography in diagnosing endocarditis in patients with MVP. Wann et al. (373) were the first to describe shaggy echoes in

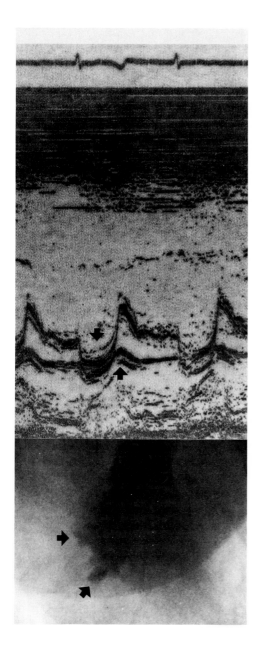

FIG. 9.15. *Case 289.* Echocardiogram and left cineventriculogram in a 68-year-old woman with floppy mitral valve proven at surgery. The patient died in the operating room as a result of dehiscence of a porcine heterograft. Chordae were intact. Note pansystolic sagging of both leaflets (*upper arrow*) and paradoxical anterior motion of the posterior leaflet in diastole (*lower arrow*). Atrial fibrillation. The left ventriculogram shows markedly irregular valve with prolapse of the middle (*upper arrow*) and posteromedial scallop of the posterior leaflet (*lower arrow*).

MVP mimicking bacterial vegetations. The prevalence of these shaggy echoes in MVP was well documented by another group (61) who noted that a sizable proportion (40%) of 85 consecutive patients with MVP had thick shaggy echoes on the mitral leaflets. With one exception, none of these patients had clinical evidence of endocarditis, either on the initial examination or on subsequent follow-up visits. The abnormal echoes were ascribed to "redundant leaflets which presented multiple surfaces for the production of echoes" (61).

ECHOCARDIOGRAPHIC DETECTION OF TRICUSPID VALVE PROLAPSE

Tricuspid valve prolapse has been demonstrated by angiography (4,143) and more recently by echocardiography (63,158,378). Chandraratna et al. (63) were the first to describe the echocardiographic features of tricuspid valve prolapse in 12 patients. They described two types of abnormalities similar to those found in MVP: posterior midsystolic motion in eight patients and a hammocklike configuration reaching a maximum in midsystole in four. These authors stressed the difficulty of echographic visualization of the tricuspid valve. In their experience, the septal leaflet is not seen echocardiographically and its prolapse can, therefore, be missed. Eight of their patients had combined mitral and tricuspid prolapse. One of their patients with floppy mitral and tricuspid valves had severe tricuspid insufficiency. A case of isolated tricuspid prolapse proven angiographically with pansystolic sagging on echocardiography was reported by Horgan et al. (158). The occurrence rate of tricuspid valve prolapse was investigated by Werner and associates (378) who found no echographic evidence of tricuspid valve prolapse in 500 consecutive patients without MVP. However, in 51 consecutive patients with MVP, 11 (21%) had associated tricuspid valve prolapse. In 11 of their patients with Marfan's syndrome, eight (73%) had MVP and of these, four (50%) had tricuspid valve prolapse.

Tricuspid valve prolapse is difficult to visualize echocardiographically, but it is not infrequent. It occurs rarely as an isolated lesion and, when present, it is usually associated with MVP. Considerable echocardiographic, angiographic, and clinical correlations are needed to define the echocardiographic criteria for tricuspid valve prolapse and their significance (123,145).

TWO-DIMENSIONAL ECHOCARDIOGRAPHY IN MVP

Two-dimensional echocardiography has added a new parameter to the diagnosis of MVP and to the understanding of its M mode echocardiographic features (138,241,289,315,316). This technique has shown that in MVP, the mitral leaflets are displaced during systole, not only posteriorly but also superiorly (Fig. 9.16) and that both leaflets are usually involved. Posteriorly displaced coaptation of the leaflets has been described as a main feature of prolapse by a group of investigators (138) while others have found excessive posterior coaptation as very common but neither sensitive nor specific (289). Systolic curling motion of the posterior mitral ring on its adjacent myocardium has also been described in MVP (138).

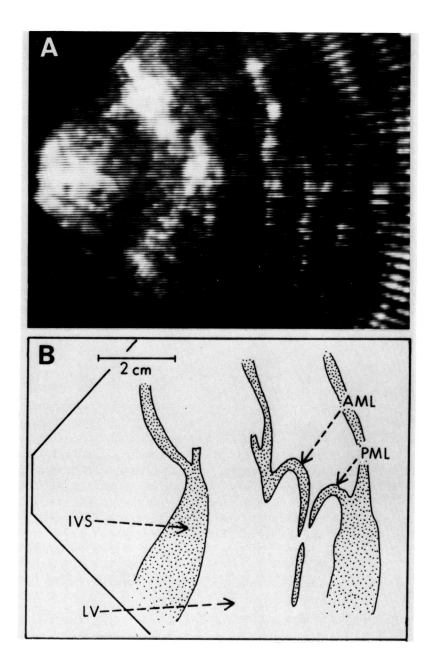

FIG. 9.16. Two-dimensional echocardiogram. Scan of a patient displaying excessive superior arching of the anterior mitral leaflet above the plane of the mitral ring. This is considered positive evidence of MVP. AML, Anterior mitral leaflet; PML, Posterior mitral leaflet; IVS, Interventricular septum; LV, Left ventricle. (From ref. 138. Courtesy of Dr. Joseph A. Kisslo. By permission of Gilbert B. W. et al. and of the American Heart Association, Inc.)

Correlation between M mode and cross-sectional echographic studies has revealed that patterns of pseudo-prolapse derive from the leaflet body. In contrast, superior–posterior prolapse, the hallmark of MVP on two-dimensional echocardiography, was associated with abnormal M mode recording from all parts of the leaflet including the free edges (316). Recording of echoes from the free edges of the leaflets has been stressed (284); to ensure this recording, apposition of the leaflets, according to some investigators, (284,316), should be demonstrated both at the beginning and at the end of systole. The same workers (316) have indicated that the free edge of the leaflet may be identified on M mode by "scanning the long and short axis until a portion of the mitral valve is encountered where the anterior and posterior leaflet echoes coapt in early systole. If the M mode is normal in this area with the transducer positioned perpendicular to the chest wall, the patient does not have prolapse." These recommendations are based on echocardiographic studies in children and require further confirmation before adopting them as a means to differentiate prolapse from pseudo-prolapse.

The exact role of cross-sectional echocardiography and the significance of its features in the diagnosis of MVP are being evaluated in various centers. It is too early to speculate on the value of this technique in the diagnosis of MVP.

ECHOCARDIOGRAPHY IN MVP: SUMMARY

Echocardiography has added a new diagnostic dimension to the diagnosis and understanding of idiopathic MVP. The M mode technique has provided most of the available information. Definite midsystolic buckling is specific of MVP. Pansystolic sagging is often the only abnormality noted in MVP with typical auscultatory and angiographic findings, but its significance as an isolated finding remains to be determined. It is not possible at this time to label sagging as a sign of valvular pathology rather than as a normal variant. Long term follow-up of patients with isolated pansystolic hammocking and documentation of complications including symptoms, arrhythmias, ruptured chordae tendineae, bacterial endocarditis, and sudden death should help establish its significance. A negative echocardiogram does not exclude the diagnosis of MVP and a positive echocardiogram, particularly in the form of hammocking, may overdiagnose this syndrome. Although cross-sectional echocardiography is most promising, its value as a diagnostic tool awaits further investigation.

Chapter 10

Radiologic Findings

In the absence of mitral regurgitation or atrial septal defect, the heart size is normal in patients with idiopathic MVP (18,84,108,175). Only 21 of my first 100 patients (175) exhibited cardiomegaly which was probably due to associated cardiac lesions in 11 of them; of the ten remaining patients, nine had angiographically proven mitral regurgitation and only one had isolated click. The cardiomegaly was minimal in four, moderate in four, and marked in the two patients who had severe mitral regurgitation requiring surgery. Left atrial enlargement was noted in only seven of the ten patients, being mild in five and marked in only the two patients who required surgery.

MITRAL VALVULAR AND ANNULAR CALCIFICATION

Calcification of the mitral cusps is infrequent in patients with MVP. Unlike rheumatic mitral insufficiency, the mitral insufficiency associated with floppy mitral valve is seldom associated with mitral valve calcification. Therefore, the detection of mitral valve calcification in patients with mitral insufficiency should favor a rheumatic etiology.

I have encountered calcification of the posterior mitral leaflet in only three patients with floppy mitral valve (175). Four other cases have been reported in the literature (54,154,197,229). At necropsy, calcification at the basal aspects of the prolapsing posterior leaflet has also been described (336); it is usually not extensive but "may be confused with calcification of the mitral ring."

When pronounced, MVP may cause added stress on the mitral annulus and may accelerate or increase the likelihood of its calcification (311). It has not been established, however, whether mitral annular calcification that is frequently seen in the elderly is a complication of floppy mitral valve. In one series of seven patients, annular calcification was noted in one patient (212) and, in another series of 13 patients (90) with severe mitral regurgitation due to floppy mitral valve, it was seen in five. At necropsy, Pomerance (278) detected mitral annular calcification in nine out of 35 cases of mucoid degeneration of the mitral valve; McKay and Yacoub (244) reported a heavily calcified mitral ring in one of their surgical patients. However, others have felt that mitral annular calcification is probably confined to the Marfan's syndrome (108,264,311). I have not noted mitral annular calcification in only two patients with MVP.

RADIOGRAPHIC APPEARANCE OF THE THORAX IN IDIOPATHIC MVP (FIG. 10.1)

Thoracic skeletal abnormalities that are frequently encountered in idiopathic MVP should be included as one of the nonauscultatory features of this syndrome, and may serve as an easily identifiable clinical indicator (38,318,322). Salomon et al. (318) defined the prevalence of these abnormalities in 24 patients with MVP. Pectus excavatum was present in 62% of the patients, "straight back" in 17%, and severe scoliosis in 8%. Eighteen of these 24 patients (75%) had a definite thoracic skeletal deformity. There was no significant difference between the male and female patients. These authors concluded that patients with these deformities should be examined clinically and perhaps by echocardiography to exclude MVP and that when murmurs are present, they should not be labeled innocent before MVP has been excluded. They postulated "that the same mesenchymal heredity that determines the skeletal habitus also affects the mitral valve, resulting in weakening and stretching of the chordae tendineae, loss of leaflet support and eventual development of prolapse of the valve leaflets."

BonTempo et al. (38), reporting on their radiologic findings in a larger series of 64 consecutive patients with MVP, have found that 72% of 50

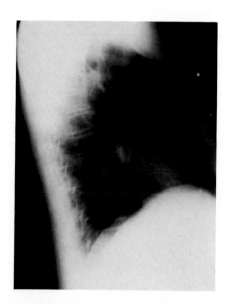

FIG. 10.1. *Case 26.* Chest roentgenogram (lateral view) in a 49-year-old man with MVP, showing a straight back. (See Figs. 8.2 and 10.1 for EKG and left cineventriculogram).

women and 78% of 14 men had an anteroposterior/transverse thoracic ratio less than the mean ratio in a normal population. Overall, 39 of the 64 patients (61%) had at least one skeletal abnormality. Scoliosis occurred in 25 subjects (39%), "straight back" in 15 (23%), and pectus excavatum in seven patients (11%). None had severe thoracic deformity. These authors provide an interesting embryologic explanation for their findings: the primordia of the mitral valve undergoes differentiation to its final form between the 35th and 42nd day of fetal development, at the time that the vertebral column and thoracic cage are beginning their chondrification and ossification. They go on to state that "any influence on growth patterns at that stage of development might affect the mitral valve and the bony thorax" (38).

Chapter 11

Hemodynamic Findings

Hemodynamic studies have been carried out on a large number of patients with idiopathic MVP with or without associated mitral insufficiency (32,91, 143,169,175,197,225,263,322,345,348,364). In general, in the absence of severe mitral regurgitation, these studies have shown no abnormalities at rest. I reported on 34 patients with MVP who underwent right and retrograde left heart catheterization and on nine who underwent only left heart catheterization (175). In this series of patients hemodynamic disturbances were generally associated with significant mitral regurgitation (Table 11.1). Of interest was the occurrence of an early diastolic dip followed by a late diastolic plateau in the left ventricular tracing in three patients, in the right ventricular tracing in three, and in both ventricles in three. The left ventricular end-diastolic pressure was found elevated in 11 out of 38 patients studied by Malcolm et al. (231). These 11 patients were not predominantly those with mitral regurgitation or significant coronary artery narrowing. A decreased cardiac compliance due to endocardial and subendocardial friction lesion (317) and to papillary muscle ischemia and fibrosis (73,364) may explain these findings.

The overall left ventricular performance was found to be normal by others (322) with normal values for functional parameters including left ventricular end-diastolic pressure, cardiac index, ejection fraction, contractility index (stroke work per end-diastolic volume) and preejection time/left ventricular ejection time (PEP/LVET). Data on the ejection fraction will be discussed in Chap. 12.

Hemodynamic abnormalities were reported by Gulotta et al. (149), who found in 20 of their 26 patients left ventricular dysfunction manifested by either elevated end-diastolic pressure, low resting cardiac index, or inappropriate rise in cardiac index during exercise. Twenty of these patients had mitral regurgitation on left ventriculography; it was mild in 11, moderate in eight, and severe in one. Correlation between mitral regurgitation and its severity and the hemodynamic abnormalities were not reported. The authors felt that the abnormal left ventricular performance cannot be ascribed to the presence of mitral incompetence in all these patients since the majority had minimal or insignificant mitral regurgitation.

Flow velocity profile studies in two patients with MVP and mitral regurgitation (189) indicated a higher percentage of ejection in the first half of systole than found in normal patients and in patients with other types of

TABLE 11.1. *Mitral regurgitation and hemodynamic disturbances in MVP*

	No. of patients	Significant MR
Elevated right atrial pressure	5	4 (80%)
Mild pulmonary hypertension	6[a]	3 (50%)
Elevated PC pressure	9	6 (67%)
Elevated LV end-diastolic pressure	9	8 (90%)
Low cardiac index	12[a]	5 (42%)

By permission of *Progr Cardiovasc Dis* 15: 623–652, 1973.
[a] Three of these patients had ASD.

mitral regurgiation; however, the aortic flow curves in one patient with MVP but no mitral regurgitation was similar to the normal patients.

Myocardial lactate abnormalities have been described in this syndrome both at rest and during pacing (111,194,261,270).

To evaluate left ventricular function in this syndrome, Kraus and Naughton (204) recorded systolic time intervals at supine rest and immediately after multistage treadmill exercise in 12 subjects with MVP. In nine subjects an increase of 1 to 49 msec was observed in LVET following exercise. They felt that exercise elicited evidence of left ventricular dysfunction.

In summary, hemodynamic studies in MVP revealed no abnormalities except in one series with high frequency of mitral regurgitation (149). Soft evidence based on echocardiography (236) and on systolic time intervals (204) has been presented to indicate impaired left ventricular performance. Further studies at rest and during exercise including hemodynamic determination, echocardiographic measurement, systolic time intervals, and gated blood pool scanning are needed for evaluation of left ventricular function in this syndrome.

Chapter 12

Angiocardiographic Findings

HISTORICAL NOTES

As the mitral valve origin of the click and late systolic murmur was being demonstrated by intracardiac phonocardiography (218,311) and by various maneuvers indicating that the late systolic murmur behaved like the murmur of mitral regurgiation (18), the angiographic counterpart of these auscultatory phenomena was described by various investigators (17,25,85,161,348). In 1962, Humphries and McKusick (161) were the first to report on cineangiography in a patient with a late systolic murmur. They described the mitral cusps as bulging back into the left atrium during systole and detected late systolic mitral insufficiency. Their published left ventriculogram in the right anterior oblique (RAO) view showed typical MVP. In the same year, Ross and Criley (312) published a left ventriculogram in the left anterior oblique (LAO) view showing typical prolapse of the posterior leaflet and late systolic mitral insufficiency in a 39-year-old male with an apical mid and late systolic murmur and nonspecific T wave abnormality. They ascribed the prolapse to ruptured chordae without surgical confirmation. Subsequently, Barlow et al. (17) described a similar left ventriculographic picture in four patients with midsystolic click and late systolic murmur and termed it "aneurysmal protrusion of the posterior leaflet of the mitral valve." The diagnostic angiographic features of MVP were described in detail by our group (171,175) and others (18,25,84,85,116,121,148,149,173,176,197, 212,292–295,322,344,348,364,380). The anatomic description of the posterior mitral leaflet as a triscalloped structure (291,295) has contributed greatly to the angiographic diagnosis of MVP and to the understanding of the angiographic features (171,175,292,293). The description of the "anterior hump sign" in the RAO view by this author (173) added a new parameter to the diagnosis of MVP. Tricuspid valve prolapse was also described subsequently (4,143,232).

The demonstration of MVP on left ventriculography provided an important diagnostic marker that assumed gradually the role of a "gold standard" (100) in the diagnosis of this syndrome. However, the specificity of the angiographic features of MVP has been questioned recently (182,340).

RADIOLOGICAL ANATOMY OF THE NORMAL AND THE PROLAPSED MITRAL LEAFLET

The anterior and posterior leaflets of the mitral valve have virtually identical surface area (308). However, the basal attachment of the posterior

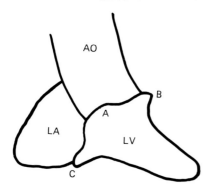

FIG. 12.1. Diagram of the left ventriculogram in prolapse of the three scallops of the posterior leaflet: Middle (A), anterolateral (B), and posteromedial (C). AO, Aorta; LA, Left atrium; LV, Left ventricle.

leaflet is twice as long as that of the anterior leaflet but the basal to margin length of the anterior leaflet is twice that of the posterior leaflet. In the left ventriculogram taken in the RAO view the two mitral leaflets are superimposed over each other and are separated by commissures at the anterosuperior and posteroinferior poles of the valve (175). In the normal heart in systole "both the mitral annulus and the mitral leaflets move toward the left ventricular cavity, not toward the left atrium" (25). In the LAO projection, the anterior leaflet occupies the medial segment of the valve ring while the posterior leaflet is on the lateral surface of the ring (312). The two leaflets can, therefore, be separated in this projection. The anterior leaflet during diastole hangs down from the aortic root to which it is attached (293). It represents a demarcation line separating the nonopacified left atrium from the opacified left ventricle and "moves like a hinged door during each cardiac cycle with its fulcrum at the aortic root" (293).

The posterior leaflet is a multiscalloped structure that is divided into three scallops: a large middle scallop and two small commissural scallops, the posteromedial and the anterolateral on either side (Fig. 12.1) (291). In the RAO view, the posteromedial scallop occupies the posteroinferior pole

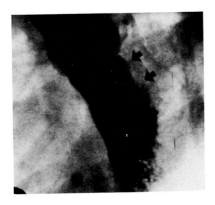

FIG. 12.2. Normal angiographic configuration of the mitral valve (in the LAO projection) that describes an almost straight line. Upper arrow points to location of anterior leaflet and lower arrow to location of posterior leaflet. The apex of the left ventricle is aligned with the aorta.

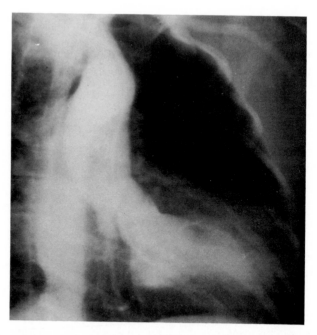

FIG. 12.3. Left ventriculogram in the left posterior oblique projection. Normal angiographic configuration of the mitral valve in a 45-year-old woman with aortic stenosis. The line of demarcation between the opacified left ventricle and the nonopacified left atrium is almost straight. There is no protrusion along the inferior pole of the valve and the anterosuperior border of the left ventricle is not interrupted by a hump.

of the valve, the middle scallop the middle portion of the valve, and the anterolateral scallop the anterosuperior pole of the valve behind the aortic root. In the LAO view the scallops of the posterior leaflet cannot be identified because of superimposition.

In the LAO view during systole the two leaflets form almost a straight line separating the left atrium from the left ventricle (Fig. 12.2). In the RAO view, during systole, the normal mitral valve forms either a straight line or a line concave toward the left atrium. Minimal "scalloping" of this line is a normal variant and should not, therefore, be considered as diagnostic of MVP. Minimal "lipping" of the posteroinferior pole of the mitral valve in the RAO view is another normal variant and is probably due to accumulation of radiopaque dye in the fornix, the small space under the mitral leaflet attachment that separates the leaflet and the left ventricle in the area of the mitral annulus (Fig. 12.3).

FREQUENCY OF PROLAPSE OF THE LEAFLETS AND OF THE THREE SCALLOPS OF THE POSTERIOR LEAFLET

Of the two leaflets, the posterior leaflet is the most commonly involved in idiopathic MVP on both anatomical and angiographic studies (175,292,

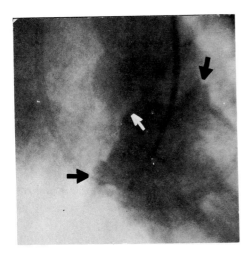 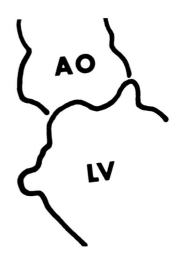

FIG. 12.4. *Case 10.* LV cine in RAO position in a 46-year-old woman. Note prolapse of middle (*white arrow*), posteromedial (*lower arrow*), and anterolateral (*upper arrow*) scallops of posterior leaflet. Moderate MR was evident. (From ref. 171. By permission)

293). In Chap. 3, I reviewed pathological evidence indicating that combined leaflet prolapse was probably the most common presentation of the MVP syndrome and that isolated anterior leaflet prolapse was uncommon. Angiographically, in a personal series of 40 patients (175), I found isolated posterior prolapse of the leaflet in 27 (posteromedial scallop in all, and middle scallop in six), isolated prolapse of the anterior leaflet in one, and prolapse of both leaflets in 12. Ranganathan et al. (293) in a study of 59 patients found similar predominance of isolated posterior leaflet prolapse that was noted in 42 patients versus prolapse of both leaflets in 17 patients and isolated prolapse of the anterior leaflet in none. Of the 42 patients, 17 had prolapse of all three scallops (Fig. 12.4) while 20 had biscalloped prolapse and five had single scallop prolapse. The posterior leaflet involvement was substantiated by morphological correlations in nine patients and by left ventriculography in the LAO projection in 24 of the 33 remaining patients.

In this series (293) as in mine (175) the middle and the posteromedial scallop prolapse appears to be an almost invariable finding. The apparently rare occurrence of prolapse of the anterolateral scallop is probably due to the difficulty in identifying this scallop in view of its superimposition over the aortic root.

PROLAPSE OF THE POSTERIOR LEAFLET

Prolapse of the middle scallop of the posterior leaflet was the first to be identified on the basis of morphologic–angiographic correlations (364), as a bulge in the midzone of the posterior leaflet in the RAO projection. The same authors (364) went on to postulate that a bulge at the posteroinferior edge of the posterior leaflet visualized in a previously published cine left ventriculogram corresponded to prolapse of the posteromedial commissural scallop. They subsequently confirmed their hypothesis by angiomorphologic correlations (292). I identified prolapse of the anterolateral scallop angiographically (171) with subsequent confirmation by the Toronto group (292) (Fig. 12.4).

RAO View

Prolapse of the posteromedial scallop produces a bulge along the posteroinferior pole of the mitral valve in the RAO projection (Figs. 12.5 to 12.7) and is undoubtedly the most difficult to identify because of the variability of the normal appearance of the mitral valve at this level. The prolapsed posteromedial scallop protrudes downward and posteriorly with a convexity toward the left atrium. It is often oval with fine serrations (Fig. 8.2) or it may point markedly downward with a configuration that has been likened to an "eagle beak" (292), a "tongue" (264) or "thumb down." I believe that it resembles a tongue or a thumb (Figs. 12.6 and 12.7) rather than an eagle beak because the latter shows initial rounding but becomes pointed, unlike the prolapsed posteromedial scallop that remains rounded. A pointed configuration on the left ventriculogram corresponds to the fornix of a normal valve rather than to a prolapsed scallop.

The middle scallop, the largest of the three, produces a central bulge (171,175,292) and its upper segment often overlaps the aortic root (Fig. 12.4).

Prolapse of the anterolateral scallop is the most difficult to visualize be-

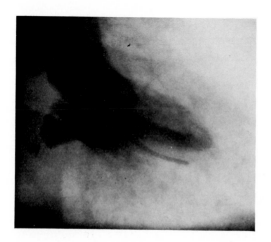

FIG. 12.5. *Case 213.* Left cineventriculogram in a 44-year-old man with intermittent midsystolic click. Note multiscalloped, prolapsed posterior leaflet, pointing downward and displaying marked convexity toward left atrium (arrow). Normal coronary arteriogram.

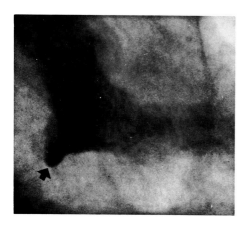

FIG. 12.6. *Case 189.* "Silent" mitral valve prolapse, involving the posteromedial scallop which resembles a tongue or a "thumb down" (*arrow*). Normal coronary arteriogram.

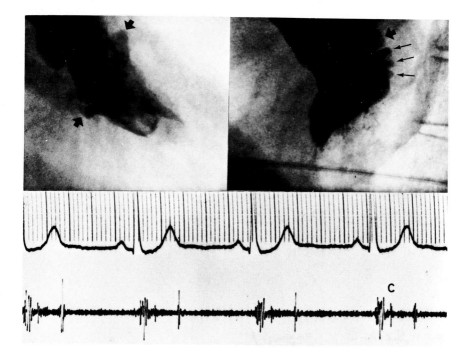

FIG. 12.7. *Case 332.* Left cineventriculogram in the RAO (A) and LAO (B) projections and phonocardiogram in a 65-year-old patient with normal coronary arteriogram. A. RAO projection. Prolapse of both leaflets. Note large anterior hump (*upper arrow*) and prolapse of the posteromedial scallop of the posterior leaflet (*lower arrow*). Increased left ventricular contractility with partial cavity obliteration. B. LA projection (hemiaxial view). Prolapse of the anterior leaflet (*upper arrow*) and of the three scallops of the posterior leaflet (*lower arrows*). The apex is aligned with the left atrium. The left ventricle and the mitral valve resembles a foot with four toes pointing toward the left atrium, the anterior leaflet corresponding to the big toe and the three scallops of the posterior leaflet to the other toes. C. Phonocardiogram showing an early to midsystolic click (C).

cause of superimposition of this scallop over the opacified aortic root. In a few cases (176,292,293) this scallop when prolapsed may protrude anteriorly, interrupting the anterosuperior border of the left ventricle or the anterior wall of the aortic root: "small hump" (176).

Visualization of the prolapsed middle and anterolateral scallop may be optimal immediately after the beginning of left ventricular injection and before becoming obscured by superimposition of the opacified aortic root. The optimal obliquity in the RAO position for visualization of prolapse is 30°. Occasionally a more oblique angulation provides a better visualization of the prolapse.

LAO View

In the LAO projection, the prolapsed posterior leaflet is noted as an irregular convexity along the inferior segment of the mitral annulus away from the aortic root (Figs. 6.11, 6.12, and 12.8). The prolapsed posterior leaflet may assume a cauliflower-like appearance (380), probably due to superimposition of scallops (Fig. 12.7).

I described in the LAO projection a round opacity, the "balloon sign" (171) that caps the hypercontracting ventricle (Figs. 12.9 and 14.9). This sign is probably due to a large mitral annulus with billowing of both leaflets through it. The LAO projection may look straight through the annulus visualizing it as a round opacity when it is markedly enlarged. I also noted multiple systolic filling defects in the LAO projection in some patients with MVP (Fig. 12.10). These filling defects probably correspond to the multiscalloped, thickened, and redundant leaflets as they fold during systole. During diastole, an unusually large nonopacified round defect is noted in the

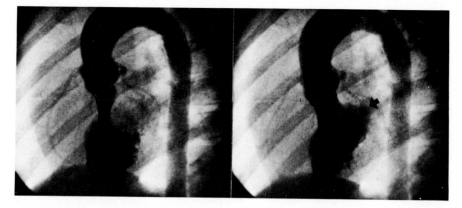

FIG. 12.8. *Case 36.* Left cineventriculogram in the lateral position in a 5-year-old girl whose ductus was divided at an earlier age. Silent prolapse of the posterior leaflet (*arrow*). A. Diastole. B. Systole.

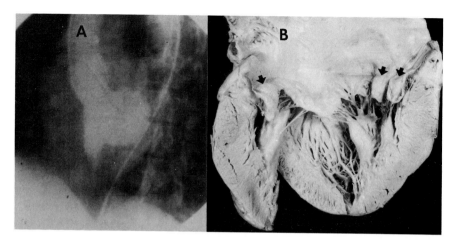

FIG. 12.9. A. Left cineventriculogram in the LAO position in a 25-year-old woman who died suddenly (Case 11 in Table 14.2). Note massive prolapse involving probably both leaflets: "balloon sign." A large mitral annulus may be a part of this angiographic appearance. B. Necropsy findings in same patient. Note "hooding" of the three scallops of the posterior leaflet (arrows) and the midanterior leaflet. The chordae are intact. (Courtesy of Drs. Jesse E. Edwards and Richard B. Guthrie).

inflow tract of the left ventricle as blood rushes from the left atrium into the left ventricle across the voluminous leaflets.

Hemiaxial view with tilting of the image intensifier 30° cephalad provides an excellent visualization of the mitral valve and a better outline of the prolapsed leaflets (Fig. 12.7), whereas in the standard LAO view there is a foreshortening of the left ventricular cavity with superimposition of the plane of the valve on the left ventricular inflow.

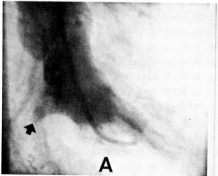
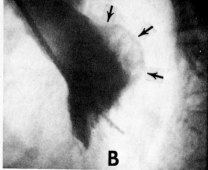

FIG. 12.10. Case 197. Left cineventriculogram in the RAO and LAO projection in a 46-year-old man. A. The RAO view is highly suggestive of MVP but may represent a normal variant. Prolapse of the postero-medial scallop of the posterior leaflet (arrow). B. The LAO projection is diagnostic of MVP, showing a large rounded protrusion of the posterior leaflet into the left atrium (arrows). Note filling defect in this protrusion, probably due to folding of voluminous and redundant leaflets. The apex of the left ventricle is aligned with the left atrium. Normal coronary arteriogram. (See Fig. 8.9 for EKG).

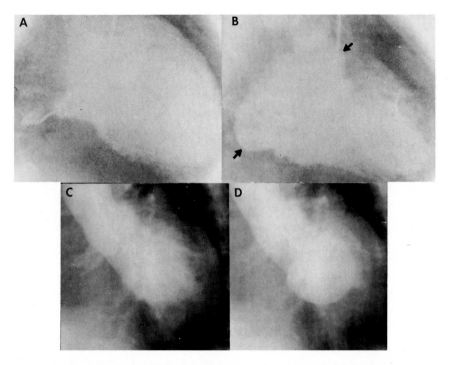

FIG. 12.11. *Case 18.* Massive mitral valve prolapse in a 46-year-old patient with midsystolic click and late systolic murmur. Five years later the patient developed sudden heart failure and a pansystolic murmur was noted. Chordal rupture is suspected. The patient has refused surgery. A. RAO view. (A, Diastole; B, Systole). Massive prolapse involving both leaflets (*arrows*). Large "doughnut" is seen in profile. B. LAO view "balloon" sign, partially due to large annulus superimposed on a foreshortened left ventricular cavity. C. Diastole. D. Systole.

PROLAPSE OF THE ANTERIOR LEAFLET

In 1972, I described the anterior "hump sign" as a sign of prolapse of the anterior leaflet in the RAO projection (173). In 50 cases without prolapse, I found the anterior wall of the left ventricle in this projection describing a smooth and uninterrupted line beneath the aortic valve. In two patients with prolapse of the posterior leaflet proven at surgery in one (Fig. 13.1) and at autopsy in one, the same smooth line was seen. However, in two patients, one with ruptured chordae tendineae to the anterior leaflet, probably superimposed on myxomatous degeneration of this leaflet (Fig. 12.12), and one with isolated prolapse of the anterior leaflet, calcification and retraction of the posterior leaflet and severe mitral regurgitation, a prominent anterior "hump" was noted (Fig. 12.13). Therefore in these two patients the posterior leaflet was not involved by myxomatous process and showed no prolapse and no redundancy on surgical exploration. In subsequent observations I noted this "hump sign" in several patients with prolapse of both leaflets demon-

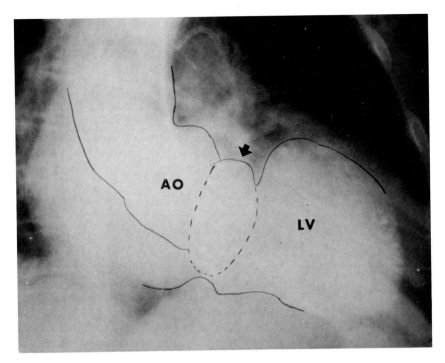

FIG. 12.12. Left ventriculogram in the left posterior oblique projection in a 54-year-old patient with myxomatous mitral valve and rupture of chordae to the anterior leaflet; the posterior leaflet was almost normal. Note anterior hump (arrow) and doughnut appearance. Severe mitral insufficiency.

strated at surgery. On the basis of these observations, I reached the following conclusions: (a) An anterosuperior "hump" in the RAO projection is an important angiographic sign of MVP and it adds confirmatory angiographic evidence to this diagnosis when prolapse along the inferior pole or the center of the valve is not evident or obvious. (b) It is a sign of prolapse of the anterior leaflet (Fig. 12.14).

Ranganathan et al. (292,293,380) and Criley et al. (84,127) have taken issue with my description, basing their conclusion on angiographic–morphologic studies (292,293) or on casts of the left ventricle in projections matching the standard angiographic projections (84). In these authors' view (Fig. 12.15), the anterosuperior hump corresponds to prolapse of the anterolateral scallop of the posterior leaflet. The casts of the left ventricle (84) were taken in patients with normal valves and do not, therefore, exclude the possibility of visualization of a prolapsed anterior leaflet as a "bulge" or "hump" along the anterosuperior border of the left ventricle in the RAO projection. The angiographic–morphologic correlations presented by Ranganathan et al. have added considerably to our understanding of the radiological anatomy of the prolapsed leaflets. However, the following criti-

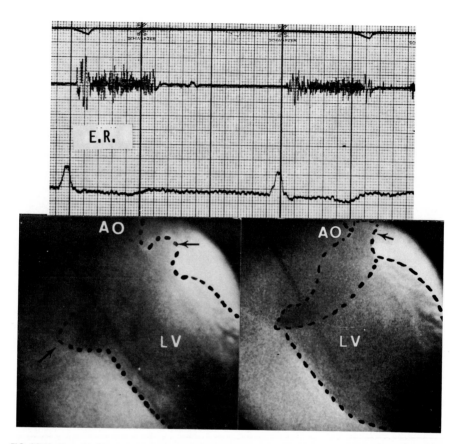

FIG. 12.13. *Case 66.* Phono and LV cineangiogram (LV cine) in the (RAO) position in a 56-year-old patient with proven prolapse of anterior mitral leaflet, retracted calcific posterior leaflet, and severe MR. Apex phono: pansystolic murmur and third heart sound. LV cine (2 frames): Prolapse of anterior leaflet, "anterior hump sign" (*upper arrow*): "posterior hump sign" (*lower arrow*), "doughnut appearance." AO, ascending aorta. (From ref. 175. By permission)

cisms can be leveled against their studies: (a) In some of their published anatomical material purporting to show isolated prolapse of the posterior leaflet additional significant involvement of the anterior leaflet was evident (176). (b) All their illustrations of anterior "hump" in isolated posterior leaflet prolapse (Fig. 2 in ref. 292 and Fig. 2 in ref. 293) actually show a minimal bulge rather than the large "hump" we have encountered in our patients with prolapse of the anterior leaflet or both leaflets (Figs. 12.16, 12.18, and 12.19). Therefore, I feel that a small "hump" interrupting the anterosuperior border of the left ventricle can be due to prolapse of the usually small anterolateral scallop of the posterior leaflet, but that a large prominent "hump" is due to prolapse of the anterior leaflet. Despite their superimposition in the RAO projection, the anterior leaflet tends to prolapse

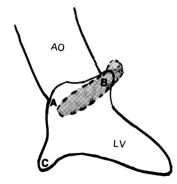

FIG. 12.14. Diagram outlining author's angiographic theory (173,175,176), RAO view, MVP. Middle scallop (A), anterolateral scallop (B) and posteromedial scallop (C) of the posterior leaflet. D. (*shaded area*) Anterior leaflet overlapping middle and anterolateral scallop, and protruding beyond the latter to form a large anterior "hump"; small anterior "hump" can be due to prolapsed anterolateral scallop of posterior leaflet.

anterosuperiorly and the posterior leaflet posteroinferiorly (175). (c) It is of interest that a published illustration of Ranganathan et al. (Fig. 4 of ref. 293) adds further confirmation to the relationship of the anterior "hump" to prolapse of the anterior leaflet. This illustration shows the RAO left ventriculogram in a patient with prolapse of both leaflets proven at surgery with a "cleft of radio-negativity separating the central bulge caused by prolapse of the anterior leaflet and postero-inferior bulge caused by prolapsed posteromedial commissural scallop of the posterior leaflet." A close look at the published angiogram shows the anterior "hump" to be a continuation of the structure marked as representing the prolapsed anterior leaflet.

The large size of the normal anterior leaflet, with further increase in its dimension when it is prolapsed, would explain the large anterior "hump" that is noted when this leaflet is involved. Despite its long basal attachment, the posterior leaflet has a small basal to margin length and, even when myxomatous, its anterolateral scallop would not account for the large anterior "hump" observed in some patients with MVP.

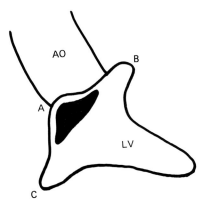

FIG. 12.15. Diagram outlining Ranganathan et al.'s (292,293) angiographic theory, RAO view, MVP. Middle scallop (A), anterolateral scallop (B), and posteromedial scallop (C) of the posterior leaflet. D. (*shaded area*) Anterior leaflet overlapping middle scallop of the posterior leaflet. AO, Aorta; LV, Left ventricle.

From a review of this controversy, I must conclude that the significance of the "anterior hump" in the RAO view as to leaflet involvement has not been established. Yet, there is general agreement that the anterior hump sign first described by this author (173,175) is an important angiographic finding that is almost diagnostic of MVP. Prior to its description, the angiographic diagnosis of MVP was made solely on the basis of changes in the middle portion and inferior pole of the mitral valve as seen in the RAO projection.

Other angiographic features indicating prolapse of the anterior leaflet have been described by Ranganathan et al. (293,294). They consist of the following: (a) "Temporal dissociation between the prolapsing leaflets with the prolapsing posterior leaflet and scallops moving toward the left atrium, first in systole, followed by a second bulge that appears centrally overlapping the prolapsed middle scallop of the posterior leaflet." In my experience, the two leaflets prolapse simultaneously and the anterior leaflet prolapses centrally and anterosuperiorly. (b) A cleft of negativity suggesting a discontinuity in outline between the prolapsing leaflets. This sign was observed in a few of my patients (Fig. 12.19) and when present is diagnostic of combined prolapse of the mitral leaflets. (c) Increased radiodensity of the central bulge as compared to the lateral bulges because the prolapsed anterior leaflet overlaps the prolapsed middle scallop of the posterior leaflet. I have not personally observed this finding and the published illustrations of this phenomenon (Fig. 5 in ref. 293) shows increased radiodensity centrally and anterosuperiorly with less density posteroinferiorly perhaps due to less opacification of the posteromedial scallop that was probably not in the path of the opaque regurgitant flow. (d) The usefulness of the LAO projection for identification of prolapse of the anterior leaflet because the two leaflets do not overlap in this view and the anterior leaflet as it prolapses remains in close proximity to the aortic root, and is seen as a convexity invading the left atrium and occupying the anterosuperior segment of the mitral annulus. I wish to confirm these findings and to stress the importance of the LAO projection.

PROLAPSE OF BOTH LEAFLETS

Prolapse of both leaflets (Figs. 12.16 to 12.19) is the most common finding in the surgical and autopsy series because of the high frequency of severe mitral regurgitation in combined prolapse. The mitral regurgitation in these patients may require mitral valve replacement or may result in congestive heart failure and death. I have just reviewed Ranganathan's description of combined leaflet prolapse. In my experience, the finding of a "doughnut sign" (175) in the RAO projection is frequently associated with combined leaflet prolapse. The mitral valve in these cases resembles a "doughnut" seen in profile (197) with the lower pole corresponding to the prolapsed posteromedial scallop of the posterior leaflet, the middle portion to the pro-

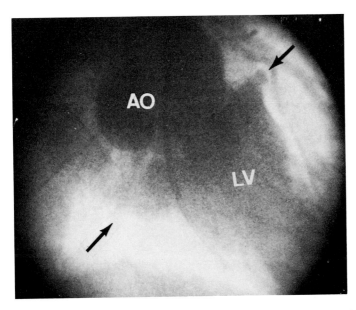

FIG. 12.16. *Case 43.* Prolapse of both leaflets in a 69-year-old man. LV cine in RAO position: Upper arrow points to "anterior hump" and lower arrow to "posterior hump." Severe MR. Coronary arteriogram was normal. See Fig. 3.2 for gross pathology and histology of MV. (From ref. 175. By permission)

lapsed middle scallop superimposed on a segment of the anterior leaflet, and the upper pole to the remaining segment of the anterior leaflet possibly overlapping the anterolateral scallop of the posterior leaflet. In massive MVP, the prolapsed leaflets in the RAO projection form a slightly irregular

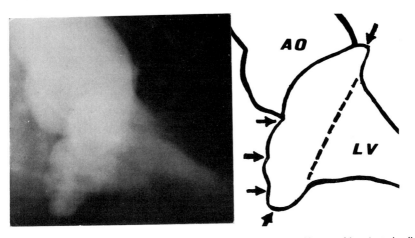

FIG. 12.17. *Case 33.* LV angiogram in the left posterior oblique position in a 62-year-old patient who died in her sleep. Poles of the doughnut-like valve are indicated by oblique arrows in diagram. Horizontal arrows point to scalloped posterior leaflet. Increased LV contractility. (From ref. 171. By permission)

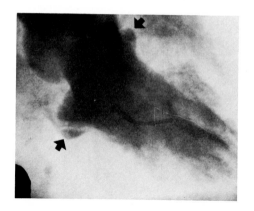

FIG. 12.18. *Case 133.* Left cineventriculo-gram in a 53-year-old man showing MVP, probably involving both leaflets. "Dough-nut" appearance. Note anterior hump *(up-per arrow)* and marked prolapse of the posteromedial scallop of the posterior leaf-let *(lower arrow).* Normal coronary arterio-gram.

round-mass protruding markedly into the left atrium, and the left ventricle, with the prolapsed leaflets at the top, resembles an "ice cream cone" (171).

MITRAL ANNULAR DILATATION IN MVP

Leachman et al. (212) attributed the angiographic appearance in MVP to a large mitral annulus and Bulkeley and Roberts (46) provided anatomic confirmation of mitral annular dilatation in idiopathic MVP. I doubt that mitral annulus per se which is usually visualized in the RAO projection in a normal heart as a straight line would account for the multiscalloped appearance of the mitral valve in MVP. The fornix beneath the annulus in a normal heart can be visualized as minimal lipping along the inferior pole of the valve or in a rare case as a small pointed anterosuperior hump. (Figs. 12.21 to 12.23) The dilated annulus may be, however, an intrinsic part of the angiographic picture if it is visualized "en face" or obliquely in the RAO view and may explain why in some patients with MVP the angiographic contour of the mitral valve does not vary significantly from systole to diastole. This finding was first noted by Leachman et al. (212) who stated that "it was noted that in each patient the diameter of the mitral valve was larger than the maximal basal diameter of the left ventricle not only during systole but also in diastole when the leaflets could not protrude toward the left atrium. The large "shadow" corresponding to the mitral valve cannot then be due only to the protruding leaflets (mainly the posterior one) but must be re-lated to the abnormally large mitral annulus." As mentioned above, annular dilatation may explain the "balloon sign" in the LAO projection. In the RAO view, the annulus may occupy the junction of the inferior hump or anterior hump and the left ventricular cavity but it is more logical to assume that the dilated annulus may be located at the tip of the humps or at variable distance from points A and B (Fig. 12.20). Inspection of the cine during systole and diastole helps locate the annulus but this is often a difficult task. The anterior and inferior humps are probably formed by leaflets protruding beyond the annulus, by the dilated annulus itself, and by a portion of the

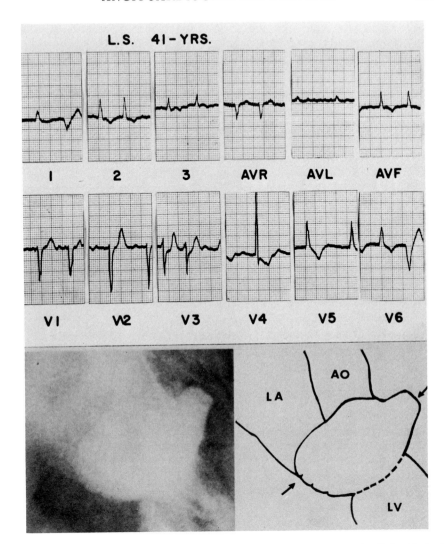

FIG. 12.19. *Case 4.* EKG and LV cine in the RAO position in a 41-year-old patient who died suddenly at age 44. The EKG shows T-wave inversion in the inferior and left precordial leads, atrial fibrillation, and multiple pvc's. LV cine shows a voluminous "doughnut" outlined by arrows in diagram. Upper arrow points to a large anterior "hump," and lower arrow to a posterior "hump." LA, Left atrium. (From ref. 171. By permission)

left ventricular inflow adjacent to the annulus. It is difficult to visualize the anterior hump, for instance, as representing the leaflet protruding beyond the superior cardiac border connecting left ventricle and left atrium and the rigid contracting myocardium. It is more logical to assume that the dilated annulus occupies the tip of the hump (B) or a point close to it, and that a segment of the hump (ABD) is a part of the left ventricular cavity and the remainder BCD is formed by the prolapsing leaflets as they abut the anterior

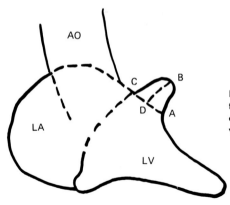

FIG. 12.20. Diagram outlining possible contribution of mitral annular dilatation to angiographic configuration in MVP. LA, Left atrium; LV, Left ventricule; AO, Aorta. (See text).

wall of the left atrium. The same reasoning would apply to the inferior hump. It is also conceivable that the "doughnut" with both humps could represent the dilated annulus seen obliquely from the side with the prolapsing scallops altering its regular contour.

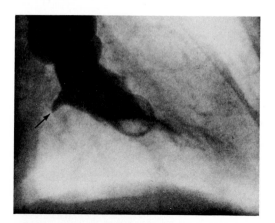

FIG. 12.21. Lipping along the inferior pole of the mitral valve (RAO view), probably corresponding to the fornix (arrow), in a patient with coronary artery disease. Normal variant.

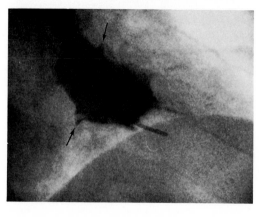

FIG. 12.22. Fornix of mitral valve (arrows). Normal variant in a patient with aortic stenosis. Note cavity obliteration.

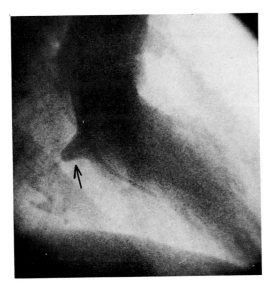

FIG. 12.23. *Case 37.* Probable normal variant in a 52-year-old man. Left cineventriculogram in the RAO projection previously reported by the author (171) as showing prolapse of the posteromedial scallop of the posterior leaflet (*arrow*). This angiographic configuration ("lipping") may be a normal variant and requires confirmation in the LAO projection or a positive echocardiogram, before making the diagnosis of MVP. (From ref. 171. By permission)

Further angiographic–morphologic correlations are needed to define the role played by the dilated mitral annulus in the angiographic configuration of MVP.

IMPORTANCE OF CINE IN THE DIAGNOSIS OF MVP

Most of the reported left ventriculographic studies in MVP have use cine techniques. Close inspection of the cine film adds considerable information that is not available on cut films and cannot be reproduced in illustrations. Popp et al. (282) described prolonged "rolling" or "inflation" of the redundant leaflets during the early phases of systole. The gradual systolic prolapse of the leaflets and their "inflation," a dynamic phenomenon, are best observed on cineangiography which allows continuous visualization of the protruding leaflets as they invade the left atrium during systole and retreat into the left ventricle during diastole. The frame by frame analysis on cineangiogram is invaluable for the demonstration of progressive prolapsing motion of the mitral valve toward the left atrium (283).

IMPORTANCE OF THE LAO PROJECTION

I stressed the importance of the LAO projection for the identification of the prolapsed leaflet. In some patients the RAO projection may show no prolapse or may show nondiagnostic or borderline abnormalities and yet the LAO projection may exhibit diagnostic changes. The converse is more common, however, and the RAO projection is usually the more diagnostic. The reason for the diagnostic dissociation of the two projections is not clear. The RAO projection should always be used and in some cases should be supplemented by the LAO projection for confirmation of nondiagnostic findings and for localization of the prolapse.

NEED FOR RIGID CRITERIA AND FOR QUANTITATION OF MVP

The description of the angiographic features in MVP has been qualitative (147,171,175,292,293) and the diagnostic criteria could be termed "ill defined and non-quantitative" (121). Because of the variability of the normal appearance of the mitral valve, there is a need for quantitation of the angiographic picture. An attempt at quantitation was reported in an abstract (121) and was based on comparison of the annulus diameter and midvalve diameter in systole and diastole. In normal valves and in valves with prominent fornix, shortening of these two axes was demonstrated whereas in MVP there was "non-shortening or actual lengthening of the systolic mitral axes." This quantitative method is promising and publication of the full article should open the way for further confirmation of these interesting data.

In the absence of quantitative criteria, the angiographic diagnosis of MVP should be made only when prolapse of the posteromedial scallop is obvious, describing a well rounded, prominent inferoposterior protrusion. This protrusion should be convex toward the left atrium. The diagnosis is strongly reinforced by the demonstration of protrusion of the middle portion of the posterior leaflet corresponding to the middle scallop. Demonstration of an anterior hump adds strong confirmatory evidence. Furthermore, the LAO projection may display clearcut abnormalities confirming the diagnosis of MVP.

ANGIOGRAPHIC PROLAPSE IN CORONARY ARTERY DISEASE

In Chap. 4, I reviewed several papers reporting on the frequency of angiographic prolapse in coronary artery disease and on the absence of auscultatory abnormalities (angioauscultatory discordance) and of echocardiographic abnormalities (angioechocardiographic discordance) in these patients. A review of our angiograms in patients with coronary artery disease has convinced me of the frequency of angiographic prolapse in these patients despite normal auscultatory and echocardiographic findings (Figs. 4.2, 4.3, and 12.24). The angiographic prolapse is usually minimal but it may be moderate or pronounced (Figs. 4.3 and 12.25). Therefore, in coronary artery disease, the angiographic demonstration of MVP is a nonspecific finding that does not add to the basic diagnosis.

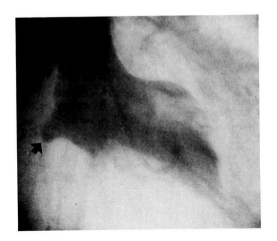

FIG. 12.24. Prolapse of the mitral valve in coronary artery disease, in the absence of a click and of echocardiographic prolapse. Note prolapse of the middle (*upper arrow*) and posteromedial (*lower arrow*) scallops of the posterior leaflet.

IS ANGIOGRAPHY THE "GOLD STANDARD" FOR THE DIAGNOSIS OF MVP?

Impressed by the abnormality of the angiographic picture in MVP, several workers (100) including this author have felt that angiography was the "gold standard" against which other diagnostic techniques should be judged. Further experience and the variability of the normal angiographic appearance of the mitral valve have convinced me otherwise. I would concur with Popp's statement that "the angiogram is not the perfect tool for diagnosing this condition" (283). The frequent occurrence of angiographic prolapse in patients with coronary artery disease, hypertrophic subaortic stenosis, and normal nonmyxomatous mitral valve have cast serious doubt on the specificity of the angiographic picture in the diagnosis of idiopathic MVP. Other workers who were originally impressed by the angiographic findings (100) have subsequently raised serious doubts as to its reliability (101). Their doubts were caused by the observation of major disagreement among 20 cardiologists and cardiovascular radiologists when they were asked to review the cineangiograms on 13 patients with obvious, equivocal, or absent MVP. The same authors concluded that it would appear that "the cineangiogram does not provide an appropriate method for the precise detection of mitral valve prolapse" (101). Similar doubts as to the reliability of angiographic diagnosis of MVP was expressed by Smith et al. (340) who analyzed the left ventricular angiograms of 336 consecutive patients and correlated them with the echocardiograms. Six of these patients had the clinical diagnosis of click-murmur syndrome and all six had angiographic prolapse of Grade 2 to 3/3 in severity. However, leaflet bulging was noted in 52 of 131 patients with ischemic heart disease (40%), 27 of 84 with rheumatic heart disease (32%), three of 19 with cardiomyopathy (16%), five of 12 with congenital heart disease (42%), and 50 of 84 with chest

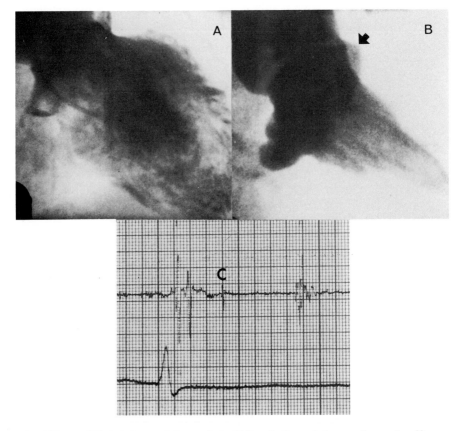

FIG. 12.25. *Case 178.* Left cineventriculogram in the RAO projection and phonocardiogram in a 62-year-old woman with severe stenosis of the left marginal circumflex artery. A. Diastole. B. Systole. Note prolapse of both leaflets, a "doughnut" sign and a large anterior hump (*arrow*). C. Phonocardiogram showing a non-ejection click (c). This case represents a coincidental occurrence of idiopathic MVP and a single vessel coronary artery disease.

pain and no significant coronary artery disease (60%). Technically satisfactory echocardiograms were available from 140 of these patients; MVP was evident on the echocardiogram of 9 (6.4%), including six with the click-murmur syndrome. These authors concluded that "some end-systolic bulging of posterior mitral leaflet scallops, therefore, is a common angiographic finding that should probably not be considered pathologic in absence of other features of the click-murmur syndrome." It should be pointed out that in the absence of click-murmur syndrome only one of their patients exhibited a Grade 3 angiographic abnormality and the great majority of their patients had only Grade I abnormality.

I believe that, in the absence of coronary artery disease or hypertrophic subaortic stenosis, a pronounced bulging of the mitral valve can be diagnostic of MVP, particularly if, in addition to the posteromedial scallop, the middle scallop is involved, a large anterior hump is noted, and the LAO projection is confirmatory. A "doughnut-like" appearance is also diagnostic. In borderline cases, auscultatory and echocardiographic confirmation is essential for an accurate diagnosis. As mentioned above, most of the difficulty in reaching an accurate angiographic diagnosis centers around the posteromedial scallop and its normal variants.

ANGIOGRAPHIC–CLINICAL CORRELATIONS

Isolated prolapse of the posterior leaflet is infrequently complicated by mitral regurgitation except when the middle scallop is involved and is often "silent" or associated with an isolated click (175). Prolapse of both leaflets is infrequently "silent" and is often associated with a late systolic or pansystolic murmur and significant mitral regurgitation (175). Ranganathan et al. (293) confirmed my finding that prolapse of both leaflets is more often associated with more severe degrees of mitral regurgitation. They also reported that triple scallop prolapse of the posterior leaflet is often associated with more severe mitral regurgitation while biscalloped and single scallop prolapse of the posterior leaflet was generally associated with a milder degree of mitral regurgitation, except when the middle scallop was involved in which case severe mitral regurgitation may occur. In their experience, a significant degree of mitral regurgitation occurring in patients with single or biscalloped prolapse probably indicates ruptured chordae to the affected scallop.

LEFT VENTRICULAR WALL MOTION ABNORMALITIES IN MVP

Reported left ventricular wall motion abnormalities in MVP were reviewed in Chap. 4. These abnormalities were not confirmed in other studies (94) that showed that no statistical difference in segmental contractility can be detected in any portion of the left ventricle when patients who have the MVP syndrome are compared to a control group of patients. In my experience, excessive emptying of the left ventricular cavity, particularly the apex, associated with prominence of the papillary muscle was evident in most patients with prolapse of both leaflets. Cavity obliteration may be noted in these patients (171,322). The ejection fraction is often increased (211,263). Abnormal systolic protrusion of the inferior wall, first described by Grossman et al. (148) and Ehlers et al. (116) was noted in other series including the author's (73,84,171,293) (Fig. 12.26). This indentation has been interpreted as either an inward pushing causing the prolapse or an inward pulling resulting from the prolapse (84). I favor the latter explanation which has been confirmed by the postoperative left ventricular angiographic studies of Cobbs et al. (73). Early relaxation of the anterior wall (293) as well as

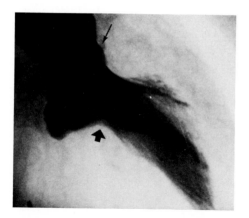

FIG. 12.26. *Case 174.* Left cineventriculo-gram in the RAO position in a 56-year-old woman with a midsystolic click (see Fig. 6.14). The three scallops of the posterior leaflet are probably involved. Note small anterosuperior hump (*upper arrow*) and buckling of the inferior wall of the left ventricle (*lower arrow*). Normal coronary arteriogram.

other wall motion abnormalities have also been described (144,148,149,179, 222,322).

In the LAO view, the apex points to the left and downward and the long axis of the left ventricle is often perpendicular to the plane of the mitral valve and is in continuity with the left atrium rather than with the aorta, as noted in normal hearts (Fig. 12.2 and 12.7). This abnormal axis has also been described in hypertrophic subaortic stenosis. The underlying cause of this axis abnormality has not been elucidated.

CORONARY ARTERIOGRAPHY IN MVP

In a review of the literature (175) published in 1973, I was able to collect 137 selective coronary arteriographic studies in MVP (18,91,95,124,144, 149,186,205,339,348,350) including 27 of my patients. This review showed that the coronary arteriogram was normal in 118, displayed slight coronary artery disease in two and significant disease in only two. Our group has studied 62 more patients for a total of 89 with the following results: normal coronary arteriogram in 79 (89%) and coronary artery disease in ten (11%). The coronary artery disease was severe (75% stenosis) in six patients, moderate (50 to 75%) in two and mild (less than 50%) in two.

Others have also reported on coronary arteriography in patients with MVP (73,211,222,226,231,263,293,332) for a total number exceeding 500 arteriograms. These studies have invariably been normal and have relegated the association of MVP and coronary artery disease to the realm of coincidence (181). The relationship of coronary artery disease and MVP was reviewed in Chap. 4 and earlier in this chapter.

A "corkscrew" or tortuous appearance of the coronary arteries (260,322) has been described and was more apparent in the branches of the left coronary artery (144). I observed this pattern frequently with or without

MVP and I concur, therefore, with Barlow et al.'s (19) statement that "its significance, if any, is uncertain." Late systolic elongation and straightening of a branch of the marginal circumflex artery that supplies the anterior papillary muscle has been described (73). This elongation contrasted with the increased angularity and moving closer together of other coronary vessels and was ascribed to late systolic elongation of the papillary muscle during buckling.

TRICUSPID VALVE PROLAPSE

Tricuspid valve prolapse (Fig. 12.27) was demonstrated by right ventriculography in a few published reports (4,143,158,231,232,322). It was first documented angiographically by the Deborah Heart and Lung Center group (143,232,322). In their second report (322) they noted tricuspid valve prolapse in 15 out of 28 cases (54%) with MVP in whom the area of the tricuspid valve ring was clearly visualized. They considered clefts and slight scalloping along the closure line of the tricuspid leaflets to be normal. The inferior cusp showed the greatest degree of prolapse into the right atrium. For optimal study of the tricuspid valve, the catheter should be positioned in the inflow portion of the right ventricle and filming should be carried out in a 15 to 25° RAO projection (143). In patients with narrow chest configuration, a more oblique view may be desirable. Hemodynamically significant tricuspid regurgitation was not detected in any of these patients. In some patients with nondiagnostic left ventriculogram, the demonstration of

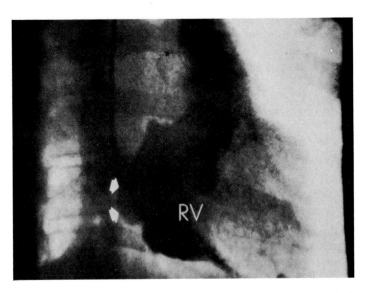

FIG. 12.27. Tricuspid valve prolapse. Right ventriculogram shows prolapse of tricuspid leaflets (arrows). (From ref. 143 By permission)

tricuspid valve prolapse on right ventricular angiography can be helpful in confirming the diagnosis of myxomatous involvement of the atrioventricular valves. This circumstance was noted in nine out of 61 patients (14.7%) reported by Maranhao et al. (232), who concluded that the identification of tricuspid valve prolapse in these patients "may allow for an explanation of chest pain and/or palpitations" (232).

The symptoms frequently seen in MVP are not modified by the association of tricuspid valve prolapse. Maranhao et al. (232) described the presence of a late systolic murmur and clicks at the left lower sternal border and their augmentation by inspiration. However, this location and the inspiratory augmentation are frequently seen in MVP alone.

As previously mentioned, Pomerance and others (54,57,193,278) noted involvement of the tricuspid valve at necropsy in a few patients with MVP. To the best of my knowledge, isolated tricuspid valve prolapse has not been reported yet.

I have not carried out right ventriculography on my patients with MVP. However, review of the published right ventricular angiograms has convinced me that the angiographic diagnosis of tricuspid valve prolapse is fraught with considerable difficulty because of the normal variability of the angiographic appearance of the tricuspid valve and ring. Only pronounced bulging beyond the tricuspid ring should be accepted as evidence of tricuspid valve prolapse. The clinical correlates of associated tricuspid valve prolapse have not been reported.

DIAGNOSTIC CONSIDERATIONS. INDICATIONS FOR LEFT VENTRICULOGRAPHY AND CORONARY ARTERIOGRAPHY IN MVP

In the majority of patients with idiopathic MVP, the diagnosis can be established by careful auscultation and by echocardiography. The auscultatory findings should be confirmed by phonocardiography. In the absence of a click, echocardiography is the only noninvasive technique available for the diagnosis of MVP. Only midsystolic buckling or pronounced pansystolic sagging of 3 to 5 mm should be accepted as echocardiographic criteria. However, echocardiography may overdiagnose this syndrome or may be false negative because of technical difficulties or the inherent deficiency of single beam approach to the complex mitral valve structure. Thus, left ventriculography would be the only diagnostic recourse in some patients. Nevertheless, it should be reserved to cases, with a nondiagnostic echocardiogram, in whom a definite diagnosis is required for psychological or therapeutic reasons. This may be the case in some patients with recurrent severe chest pain associated with ST-T abnormalities who are frequently admitted to the hospital, and even monitored in the coronary care unit. Some of these patients are convinced that they have coronary artery disease and become "emotional cripples"; their physician finds it impossible to rule out this disease. A stress test is often not helpful because "ischemic" ST-T changes can be recorded in idiopathic MVP. A negative thallium stress test should be most reassuring but further studies are needed to confirm its value. A recent study (198,240) would indicate that a negative exercise perfusion scintigram makes the presence of coronary artery disease unlikely and "may, therefore, obviate the need for invasive studies" (240). However, doubt as to the value of stress scintigraphy has been raised (248,268). In these patients, left ventriculography in conjunction with coronary arteriography are indicated to alleviate anxiety and a negative study would have a beneficial effect on chest pain. The physician is also reassured by the absence of coronary disease and repeated hospital admissions are avoided.

Angiographic studies are particularly indicated in patients with exertional chest pain and in those harboring risk factors for coronary artery disease. As mentioned previously, coronary artery disease and idiopathic MVP can coexist in the same patient and finding of a click and a positive echocardiogram, although diagnostic of idiopathic MVP, do not rule out associated coronary artery disease.

Left ventriculography on coronary arteriography should be carried out in patients with advanced MVP and severe mitral insufficiency (e.g., the "floppy mitral valve syndrome"). In these patients, only a pansystolic murmur is heard and MVP can be suspected if a click had been heard in the past, but this is an uncommon finding in these patients. Echocardiography is most helpful in differentiating MVP from rheumatic mitral insufficiency and hypertrophic subaortic stenosis. However, left ventriculography and coronary arteriography are indicated if the mitral insufficiency is pronounced and the associated symptoms are severe enough to require surgical consideration.

Left ventriculography is also indicated in patients with secundum atrial septal defect undergoing cardiac catheterization. Associated MVP is frequent in these patients (180,371) and is often evident by auscultation and echocardiography. However, the MVP may be silent and the echocardiogram nondiagnostic or technically poor. In such cases, left ventriculography is recommended, particularly if the left ventricule can be readily entered when the saphenous venous approach is used.

Chapter 13

Associated Diseases

In attempting to explain the etiology and various features of idiopathic MVP, it is natural that association with other diseases should be sought. It is hoped that this association may provide the missing parts needed to put together the "jigsaw puzzle" presented by this fascinating entity (264). Unfortunately, the high prevalence of MVP would be expected to result in a high probability of chance occurrence with other disorders in the same subject. The rush to publish any association and to term it causal and etiological has confused the issue and has probably hampered research in this syndrome. The diseases most commonly associated with MVP are coronary artery disease, rheumatic heart disease, and systemic inherited connective tissue disorders such as Marfan's syndrome, Ehlers-Danlos syndrome, and so forth. Hypertrophic subaortic stenosis and secundum atrial septal defect should also be added. In previous chapters I presented evidence to indicate that the association of MVP, coronary artery disease, and rheumatic heart disease is probably casual rather than causal. These two diseases will not be discussed in this chapter.

INHERITED CONNECTIVE TISSUE DISORDERS

The close association of Marfan's syndrome and mitral valve prolapse was reviewed in Chap. 4.

MVP in the Ehlers-Danlos Syndrome

The Ehlers-Danlos syndrome is an uncommon heritable disorder of connective tissue characterized by fragility and hyperextensibility of the skin, hypermobility of the joints, bleeding, and a variety of visceral abnormalities. MVP often associated with mitral insufficiency has recently been reported in this syndrome, particularly in type III which is known as the joint hypermobility type with minimal skin hyperextensibility and other cutaneous manifestations (247). In one series of 45 patients (6), six were found to have papillary muscle dysfunction, which is probably a misnomer for MVP. A higher prevalence of MVP (nine out of 11 patients) was reported in a recent comprehensive study (50) utilizing clinical evaluation, echocardiography (11 patients) and angiography (six patients). MVP was an isolated cardiac lesion in four patients but it was associated with tricuspid valve prolapse or with shunt lesions in the remaining five. The published left ventricular angiogram in one case (40) was diagnostic of marked MVP with mitral regurgitation in the absence of coronary artery disease; a pansystolic murmur and paroxysmal atrial tachycardia were also reported in this patient. In another case (49) of type III Ehlers-Danlos syndrome, a loud systolic click followed by a late systolic murmur were heard and right bundle branch block and left anterior hemiblock were noted.

The mitral valve involvement in Ehlers-Danlos syndrome is more important than previously acknowledged (49) and its high frequency rules out a chance association. Therefore, patients with Ehlers-Danlos syndrome should be evaluated by auscultation and echocardiography for associated MVP and patients with MVP should be investigated for underlying Ehlers-Danlos syndrome by close examination of skin and joints.

MVP in Osteogenesis Imperfecta

Osteogenesis imperfecta is characterized by blue sclerae, skeletal abnormalities, deafness, poor teeth, and multiple fractures. Aortic insufficiency is the most common valve lesion, but mitral valve disease has been described in a few reports (87,157,351,374,391). Mitral valve aneurysm with marked decrease in fibrous connective tissue was reported in a 50-year-old man (87). Two other cases of redundant mitral valve leaflets, dilated mitral annulus, and ruptured chordae tendineae (391) underwent mitral valve replacement with the expected postoperative hemorrhage. In three other reported cases (351,374) of severe mitral insufficiency, the mitral valve ring was dilated, the mitral valve showed severe myxomatous degeneration in one patient (351), was "floppy" with elongated fragile chordae in the second (374), and showed ruptured chordae tendineae in the third (351). It is possible that echocardiographic studies in patients with osteogenesis imperfecta would demonstrate a prevalence of MVP as high as that observed in Marfan's syndrome (43,351).

MVP in Inherited Disorders of Metabolism

Cardiac involvement in inherited disorders of metabolism was the subject of a recent review article (35) that pointed out that the mitral valve was the most commonly affected valve in these disorders, and that mitral insufficiency was often present. Floppy mitral valve has also been described in pseudoxanthoma elasticum (306).

Disorders of Carbohydrate Metabolism

Mitral valve involvement is common in mucopolysaccaridosis occurring in about 70% of patients with Hurler's and Hunter's syndrome. Clinical mitral insufficiency is a predominant feature and the mitral valve exhibits fibrosis and nodule formations but not the redundancy noted in patients with idiopathic MVP, Marfan's syndrome, Ehlers-Danlos syndrome, and so forth. However, a case of Sanfillipo syndrome with thick free edge of the anterior leaflet prolapsing into the left atrium was reported.

Disorders of Protein Metabolism

No mitral valve abnormality reminiscent of MVP has been reported.

Disorders of Lipid Metabolism

Mitral insufficiency and interchordal hooding of the mitral valve have been reported in Fabry's disease and redundancy and hooding of the mitral valve have also been described in Sandhoff's disease (34,35). Histologically, the mitral valve was thickened by fibrous and myxoid tissue.

MVP IN CONGENITAL HEART DISEASE

The occurrence of MVP in association with congenital heart disease has been described. Of all types of congenital heart disease, secundum atrial septal defect has been the lesion most closely associated with MVP and most stressed in the literature.

MVP and Secundum Atrial Septal Defect

The association of MVP with secundum atrial septal defect (ASD) (Figs. 13.1 and 13.2) has been described in numerous articles (19,80,154,180,192, 229,243,267,353,370,371). It was first noted by Pocock and Barlow (80) and McDonald et al. (187). Altogether more than 200 cases of this association have been reported including 10 cases in my series.

Analysis of left ventricular angiogram by Betriu et al. (29) in 54 patients with secundum ASD gave evidence of MVP in 20 (37%), but echocardiography was not performed in this series. In nine of these 20 patients (45%), there was no clinical evidence of a mitral lesion; thus the rate of unsuspected MVP with secundum ASD was 20% (nine of 43 patients), confirming the frequency of "silent" MVP that we had previously reported (169,175,178). In 11 patients (20%) there was clinical evidence of a mitral valve lesion (pansystolic murmur in nine and midsystolic click in two, one of whom had a late systolic murmur). Twelve of the 20 patients with MVP suffered from chest pain, five patients had T wave inversion in the inferior leads, and four in the left precordial leads. Others (213) studying prospectively 92 patients with secundum ASD aged 15 to 69 years, documented MVP by clinical or angiographic evidence in 16 (17%), whereas a third

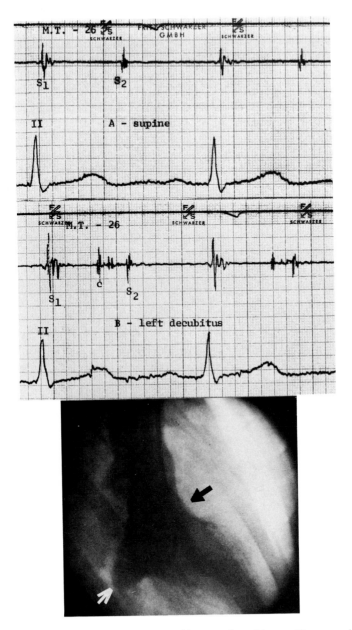

FIG. 13.1. Case 56. MVP and ASD. Midsystolic click (c) recorded in a 26-year-old woman only in the left decubitus position. The left cineventriculogram shows prolapse of posteromedial scallop of posterior leaflet (*lower arrow*) and no mitral regurgitation. The anterior wall of LV is not interrupted by a "hump" (*upper arrow*). ASD and prolapse of the posterior leaflets were proven at surgery. (From ref. 175. By permission)

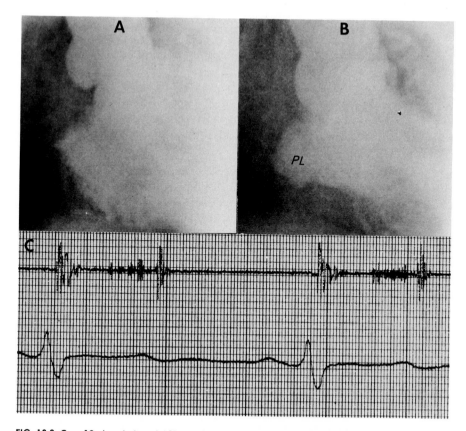

FIG. 13.2. *Case 19.* Association of ASD and MVP in a 64-year-old woman. A. Left cineventriculogram in diastole. B. Left cineventriculogram in systole showing prolapse of the posteromedial scallop of the posterior leaflet (PL). C. Apex phonocardiogram showing multiple clicks and a late systolic murmur.

group (187) reported a prevalence of 41% (19 out of 46). However, the latter group has included 12 angiograms, carried out through left atrial, right ventricular, or pulmonary artery injections, which do not provide adequate visualization of the mitral valve.

The prevalence of secundum ASD in series reporting primarily on MVP has been much lower since idiopathic MVP is a much more common lesion than ASD. For instance, in one series (80) of 200 patients with a late systolic murmur or nonejection click, 17 patients (8.5%) had an associated ASD, and in another series (89) of 50 patients with MVP six had ASD (12%). In my own series of 350 patients with MVP, I noted secundum ASD in 10 (3%).

In most of the reported cases of this association, the diagnosis of MVP was based on left ventricular angiography and an inordinately high frequency of "silent" MVP was reported (29,187,243,370). Echocardiography was performed in only one series (267) and was diagnostic of MVP in 30% (eight of 26) of patients with atrial septal defect. On auscultation, a pansystolic murmur has been more frequent than a late systolic murmur and, except in one series (80), midsystolic clicks have been relatively infrequent (213).

The association of secundum ASD with MVP is greater than can be accounted for by chance (177). Idiopathic MVP is a prevalent mitral valve disorder; however, its prevalence in ASD (17.2%) is higher than in the general population. Moreover, in no other congenital heart lesion has MVP been encountered with such high frequency. In VSD, for example, the association of MVP is extremely rare (243). A partial explanation for the high frequency of "floppy" mitral valve noted at surgery in ASD may be the relative ease of visual observation of the mitral valve in ASD as opposed to other congenital anomalies.

Doubt has been raised as to the true frequency of this association, particularly since most of the reported cases based the diagnosis on left ventricular angiographic findings. Schwartz et al. (327) in a study of 55 patients with ASD have pointed out that the appearance of the mitral ring on left ventriculogram in secundum ASD may lead to an erroneous diagnosis of MVP without clinical or echocardiographic substantiation. However, the presence of a nonejection click, the auscultatory "hallmark" of MVP, has been documented in a large number of patients with ASD (80,213,353,370), redundant myxomatous mitral valve leaflets were observed in 33 of them (29, 56,164,192,243,252,370) and the published angiogram (29,187,192,213, 243,370) have been quite diagnostic of prolapse.

Future studies of this association should use stringent angiographic criteria. It is possible that the left ventricular angiogram (327) in ASD may exhibit a normal variant reminiscent of mild MVP and due either to appearance of the mitral ring, prominence of the fornix, or to the relative small size of the left ventricle (68). In the presence of this minimal deformity and in the absence of a click, the diagnosis of MVP should only be made if the echocardiogram is confirmatory. There is a need for echocardiographic evaluation of a consecutive series of patients with ASD to provide additional data on the true prevalence of MVP in this lesion.

It is not unusual to have the surgeon report a normal mitral valve in atrial septal defect despite auscultatory, echocardiographic, or angiographic evidence of MVP. It may be impossible with a nonbeating empty heart to visualize the dynamic abnormality of prolapsing mitral cusps (243), particularly if only one or two scallops of the posterior leaflet are involved.

From a diagnostic viewpoint, midsystolic click-late systolic murmur and pansystolic murmur should be diligently sought in all patients with ASD, particularly in the presence of ST-T changes in the inferior leads and of ventricular arrhythmias. Echocardiography should be performed not only to help diagnose ASD but also to search for associated MVP. During surgical closure of ASD, the surgeon should inspect the mitral valve for MVP. Conversely, signs of ASD should not be overlooked in patients with MVP. Some workers (89) reported physiological rather than the typical fixed splitting of the second sound in ASD associated with MVP. However, this atypical auscultatory finding has not been reported by others. In uncomplicated MVP, the occurrence of "straight back" and pectus excavatum may result in physical, electrocardiographic, and radiographic signs that erroneously suggest associated ASD (38,108). Echocardiographic examination of right ventricular size and septal motion should clarify the diagnosis.

Some workers (370) have recommended that every patient with ASD should have a left ventriculogram whenever the left ventricle can be readily entered via the ASD and the mitral valve such as in saphenous venous approach (180). However, if the venous catheterization is carried out through the arm and the catheter cannot be readily advanced into the left ventricle, retrograde left ventricular catheterization via the brachial artery is not warranted because the information provided by auscultation and echocardiography would be sufficient to make the diagnosis of MVP. In the presence of a pansystolic murmur, left ventriculogram should be performed regardless of the catheterization technique needed to gain access to the left ventricle. In the differential diagnosis of mitral regurgitation associated with ASD, MVP should be added to ostium primum defect, cleft mitral valve in the absence of a primum defect, and rheumatic heart disease. Left axis deviation, the electrocardiographic "hallmark" of ostium primum defect, can also be found in combined ASD and MVP (177,243,370,371) and does not, therefore, separate these two entities. The angiographic and echocardiographic features are distinct.

The prognostic and therapeutic implications of this unexplained association are worth mentioning. In isolated ASD, surgical closure would result in complete "cure" of the disease. However, no such result can be promised in the presence of MVP, an entity with an uncertain outlook. The prognosis is particularly guarded in the presence of mitral insufficiency as evidenced by a late systolic or a pansystolic murmur (213,253). In some of these patients, mitral insufficiency may be severe enough to require mitral annuloplasty or mitral valve replacement as was the case in nine patients reported in one prospective series (213). Chordal rupture can complicate the picture (80,213) and was reported to have occurred 2 to 3 years later in four patients with ASD, MVP, and mitral insufficiency who had intact chordae on the first operation for closure of an ASD (213). In only one of these patients was chordal rupture due to bacterial endocarditis. Symptoms due to MVP (e.g., chest pain, palpitations, dyspnea) can be disabling and would alter the prognosis. Arrhythmias and the rare occurrence of sudden death can also complicate the picture when MVP is associated with ASD. Moreover, infective endocarditis, an unheard of complication of isolated secundum ASD, can occur in MVP, particularly when mitral insufficiency is present.

Antibiotic prophylaxis, which is not warranted in isolated ASD and in "silent" MVP and which is of questionable indication in isolated click, is definitely indicated when ASD is associated with MVP, late systolic or pansystolic murmurs.

Although the association of ASD and MVP which is greater than can be accounted for by chance is not yet understood embryologically, it would suggest a developmental abnormality of the mitral valve (80). The association of MVP, ASD, and Holt-Oram syndrome has been reported (180). This interesting case bridges two common associations, Holt-Oram syndrome and ASD with MVP and ASD. It also adds further support to the concept that MVP is not necessarily an isolated cardiac disorder but "on occasion may be part of a more generalized heritable disorder of connective tissue" (180).

To explain the association of MVP and ASD other workers (267) postulated traumatic myxomatous degeneration resulting from pulmonary venous flow being deflected from the septum primum into the mitral leaflets. I believe that this hypothesis is unlikely. It is possible that in a few patients the association of MVP and ASD can be explained by the left atrial effect of the associated mitral regurgitation that may distend the valvular competent foramen ovale (336). A similar mechanism has been postulated for some cases of associated ASD and mitral stenosis.

A recent abstract (62) has reported the association between ASD and tricuspid valve prolapse. Tricuspid valve prolapse was noted on echocardiography performed in 52 patients with ASD of whom three had associated MVP.

MVP in Other Congenital Heart Anomalies

MVP has been described in various types of congenital heart disease but its prevalence has been low, suggesting a coincidental rather than a true association.

As mentioned above, MVP is rarely associated with ventricular septal defect (187) except in one series that reported a 7.5% prevalence (3 out of 40) but based the diagnosis of MVP on left ventriculograms that were not always selective. Even in this latter series, the 7.5% prevalence of MVP in ventricular septal defect was close to its prevalence in the general population. Five patients with other forms of congenital heart disease were encountered in a series of 200 cases of MVP (80): one case of Eisenmenger's syndrome due to ventricular septal defect and four cases of patent ductus arteriosus. In our series of 350 patients with MVP we encountered one patient with aorticopulmonary window, one with patent ductus arteriosus, two with small ventricular septal defect, and one with mild pulmonary infundibular stenosis.

MVP with considerable "hooding" has been described in two of five specimens of hearts from patients with supravalvular aortic stenosis (23). It has also been noted echocardiographically in one patient with membranous subaortic stenosis complicated by aneurysm of the membranous septum (59). In another case (168) myxomatous transformation of the aortic and mitral valve was associated with a nonobstructive "sail-like" membrane.

Prolapse of the mitral valve was described in three patients with Ebstein's anomaly of the tricuspid valve (63,307); "floppy" mitral valve was evident at necropsy in one of these patients (307). As pointed out by Roberts (307), one of the major characteristics of Ebstein's anomaly is a striking redundancy of the tricuspid leaflets, but the caudal displacement of these leaflets prevents their systolic prolapse into the right atrium. Left ventriculography in Ebstein's anomaly would probably unmask a higher prevalence of MVP than has been hitherto noted. Corrected transposition, which can be associated with Ebstein's anomaly of the left atrioventricular valve, was reported to be associated with both mitral and tricuspid prolapse in the absence of Ebstein's anomaly (79). This represents, in all likelihood, a coincidental occurrence.

Association of MVP with Uhl's anomaly (idiopathic right ventricular myocardial hypoplasia with right ventricular dilatation) has been described in two cases (107,131).

Bharatan and Lev (30) described in 36 patients congenital polyvalvular disease with involvement of all valves in a dysplastic process. The A-V valve leaflets were redundant and all valves exhibited an increase in spongiosa and a "copious" infiltration with acid mucopolysaccharides reminiscent of changes described in myxomatous mitral valve. These changes were associated with congenital heart disease in 33 cases: 16 with a shunt, five with intracardiac obstruction, and 12 with a combination of obstruction and shunt. Of interest was the occurrence of ASD in 20 of 28 cases with shunt. This study confirmed the frequency of association of MVP and ASD. Other types of congenital heart disease reported in this series included ventricular septal defect, patent ductus arteriosus, coarctation, pulmonic stenosis, and so forth. These cases were often associated with trisomy 18 or trisomy 13–15.

MVP has been reported in association with Turner's syndrome in four cases (32,99,154,202) and with Noonan's syndrome (Turner phenotype with normal chromosome pattern) in one case (361). These two cases represent, probably, a random association.

ASSOCIATION OF MVP AND IDIOPATHIC HYPERTROPHIC SUBAORTIC STENOSIS

Several reports have described the association of MVP and idiopathic hypertrophic subaortic stenosis (IHSS) (18,58,65,84,105,170,356,365), two entities that have aroused considerable interest recently. The evidence in favor of such association and the etiological connection postulated by some workers may be summarized as follows.

Angiographic Evidence

In 1971, having reviewed the left ventriculogram in my series of 22 cases of IHSS (170), I was impressed by the frequency of ballooning or prolapse of the posterior mitral leaflet in this entity [15 of 22 cases (68%)]. I felt that the prolapse of the posterior leaflet past the anterior leaflet was due to the reduction of left ventricular end systolic volume in IHSS. I further postulated that "the reduced end systolic volume, by narrowing the distance between the papillary muscle and the mitral leaflet, permit the latter to billow into the left atrium before tensing of the chordae could check its advance" (Figs. 13.3 to 13.5). I termed this prolapse secondary as opposed to primary MVP, the more common type which is due to myxomatous transformation of the mitral valve. I also felt that secondary MVP may be one of the mechanisms responsible for mitral regurgitation in IHSS (170). The anterior mitral leaflet is not subjected to the mechanism I postulated because it has been shown angiographically and echocardiographically that this leaflet moves anteriorly during systole in IHSS (Fig. 13.4). The mechanism of the anterior motion has been ascribed to either a Venturi effect or to septal hypertrophy, anterior displacement of the anterior papillary muscle, and abnormal pull on the leaflet. The abnormal posterior leaflet motion in IHSS may also be due to the systolic anterior motion of the anterior leaflet causing distortion of normal systolic apposition ("keystone effect") of the two mitral

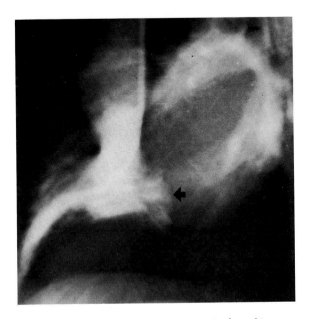

FIG. 13.3. Angiographic prolapse of a multiscalloped posterior leaflet (arrow) in a young man with proven IHSS. (From ref. 170. By permission.)

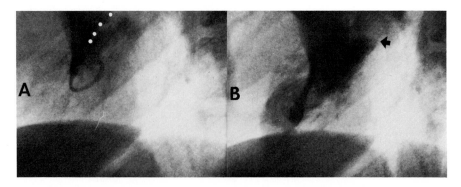

FIG. 13.4. Angiographic MVP in IHSS in an 18-year-old boy. **A.** Left cineventriculogram in the LAO projection—anterior systolic motion of the anterior leaflet, outlined with dotted lines. **B.** In the same projection, prolapse of the posterior leaflet (arrow) is noted.

leaflets, thereby permitting the posterior leaflet to prolapse during systole (59). Others (365) have theorized that the asymmetric myocardial hypertrophy in IHSS could result in inequality of functional length of some chordae and partial prolapse of the mitral leaflets.

Whatever its mechanism, the posterior leaflet prolapse in IHSS is only an angiographic finding that is not associated with myxomatous degeneration of the mitral valve, nonejection clicks, or with echocardiographic evidence of prolapse. This angiographic prolapse is nonspecific and its finding should not be used to implicate IHSS in the etiology of idiopathic MVP. My article (170), unfortunately, has been misquoted as implying such etiological correlation (see Chap. 4). It is possible that the secondary MVP may be one of the mechanisms responsible for mitral regurgitation in IHSS.

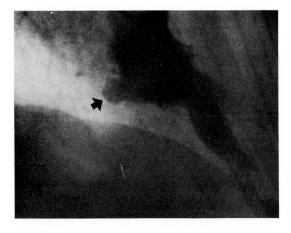

FIG. 13.5. Angiographic prolapse of the posterior leaflet in IHSS. Left cineventriculogram in the RAO projection. Arrow points to the prolapsed posteromedial scallop of the posterior leaflet.

Auscultatory Evidence

As I have just mentioned, a midsystolic click was not a feature in our patients who had IHSS and secondary angiographic prolapse of the posterior leaflet (170) and in more than 100 cases of IHSS seen by our group since publication of my editorial. Others (105,250,365) reported the association of IHSS and nonejection clicks in seven patients. In one series (365) of 90 patients with hypertrophic obstructive cardiomyopathy, four patients (4.4%) presented with a click that was early in two and midsystolic in two, but this prevalence is close to that of MVP in the general population. Therefore, a casual association between IHSS and midsystolic click can be postulated on the basis of the relatively infrequent occurrence of nonejection click in IHSS.

A pseudoejection sound in IHSS has been described (356) and has been ascribed to sudden halting of the systolic anterior motion of the anterior leaflet as demonstrated by echophonocardiographic correlations. This sound was detected in 10 of 23 patients with IHSS (356), was low or medium pitched in all but two, and was related to the severity of the left ventricular outflow obstruction. It followed the onset of the Q wave by 150 to 230 msec and the first heart sound by 70 to 150 msec and was definitely earlier in systole than the nonejection click seen in idiopathic MVP. Unlike the aortic ejection sound, this pseudo ejection sound followed the upstroke of the indirect carotid pulse by 40 to 100 msec and occurred near its peak. Although the authors have presented evidence to correlate the sound with the SAM of the anterior leaflet, it should be pointed out that MVP can be associated with early nonejection clicks (163,260).

Echocardiographic Evidence

To the best of my knowledge, echocardiographic prolapse of the posterior leaflet as opposed to systolic anterior motion of the anterior leaflet has never been demonstrated in IHSS. I have not noted asymmetric septal hypertrophy in my series of MVP; however, an unusually high prevalence of asymmetric septal hypertrophy in MVP (16 out of 190) was demonstrated in a recent study (65). The diagnosis of MVP in these 190 patients was made by means of echocardiography, and all 16 patients who had asymmetric septal hypertrophy had the classic midsystolic buckling, and none had SAM; a nonejection click was noted in nine of these 16 patients. The ratio of thickness of the interventricular septum to that of the posterior wall was 1.5 or greater in all patients. The significance of these observations is not clear and further confirmation by other workers is needed. Although asymmetric septal hypertrophy is the most common echocardiographic finding in obstructive cardiomyopathy, it has also been described in other entities (65).

Low amplitude systolic humps reminiscent of those seen in IHSS have been described in a few cases of MVP (39,145,280) and can be termed pseudo-SAM. They are probably due to systolic anterior motion of chordae tendineae (289) or to superimposition of echoes derived from the anterior portion of the mitral annulus (315). These humps have not been correlated with clinical, hemodynamic, angiographic, or other echocardiographic evidence of IHSS.

Pathological Evidence

Only one case of association of IHSS with marked myxomatous transformation of the mitral valve has been reported (150), indicating a random association of these two entities. The patient was 69 years old and presented with a loud pansystolic murmur but no click. The echocardiogram showed prominent SAM and asymmetric septal hypertrophy. At necropsy, asymmetric septal hypertrophy and a small left ventricular cavity were demonstrated. The posterior mitral leaflet was thickened and had "focal areas of myxomatous billowing between some of the chordal insertions." No evidence has been presented yet to indicate that the prolapse of the posterior leaflet in IHSS that is noted on left ventriculography is associated with secondary development of myxomatous degeneration of this leaflet.

In summary, angiographic demonstration of MVP is not uncommon in IHSS. No posterior motion of the posterior leaflet has been demonstrated by echocardiography. The occasional report of association of proven IHSS with a nonejection click or with myxomatous mitral valve is probably due to chance occurrence of two common entities.

Differential Diagnosis Between MVP and IHSS

MVP and hypertrophic subaortic stenosis share many clinical, auscultatory, and angiographic features that can confuse the differential diagnosis between these two diseases (Tables 13.1 and 13.2). Both entities are associated with various symptoms including chest pain, dyspnea, palpitations and, more commonly in IHSS, occurrence of sudden death. The nonejection click is a distinctive feature of MVP and, if detected in a patient with IHSS, would indicate casual association of both entities. An early click, however, can be heard in IHSS and MVP and in both a late systolic or pansystolic murmur with late systolic accentuation can be heard. Response of the intensity of the murmur to various maneuvers (squatting, upright position, passive leg raising) is usually similar in these two diseases except that with Valsalva maneuver, the murmur becomes louder in IHSS but longer and not necessarily louder in MVP. However, in some forms of IHSS with severe fixed obstruction, the murmur may decrease in intensity with Valsalva maneuver (58). With amyl nitrite inhalation, the murmur becomes louder in both entities but in MVP early softening of the murmur is observed (9). The

TABLE 13.1. *Idiopathic hypertrophic subaortic stenosis (IHSS) versus idiopathic MVP*

	IHSS	MVP
Pathology	Septal hypertrophy—disarray of myocardial fibers	Myxomatous transformation of the mitral valve
Symptoms		
Chest pain	Yes	Yes
Dyspnea	Yes	Yes
Palpitations	Yes	Yes
Sudden death	Yes	Yes
Auscultatory findings		
Early click	In a few patients (pseudo ejection sound)	In a few patients
Mid–late systolic click	No	Yes
Late systolic murmur	Occasionally	Often
Midsystolic murmur	Frequent	Uncommon
Pansystolic murmur	Yes in the presence of mitral regurgitation	Yes, in the presence of moderately severe to severe mitral regurgitation
Response of murmur to maneuvers		
Standing	Increases	Increases and occurs earlier
Squatting	Decreases	Decreases and occurs later
Valsalva	Increases	Becomes longer but not necessarily louder
Amyl nitrite	Increases	Increases after initial softening
Electrocardiogram		
Arrhythmias	Yes	Yes
Preexcitation	Yes	Yes
LVH	Yes	No
Echocardiographic features		
Septal hypertrophy	Yes	No, except in one series (65)
Pansystolic hammocking or midsystolic buckling of posterior leaflet	No	Yes
SAM	Yes	No, except for occasional small Hump
Left ventricular angiogram		
Cavity obliteration	Yes	Yes
Apex pointing anteriorly in the LAO view	Yes	Yes
V shaped filling defect	Yes	No
Prolapse of posterior leaflet	Yes	Yes
Prolapse of anterior leaflet	No	Yes
Mitral regurgitation may occur	Yes	Yes
Radiology		
Cardiomegaly if severe mitral regurgitation	Yes	Yes
Cardiomegaly in the absence of LVH by ECG may occur	No	Yes
Coronary arteriogram	Normal, large arteries	Normal
Prognosis	Guarded	Generally good
Ruptured chordae tendineae	Most uncommon	Not infrequent
Bacterial endocarditis	Yes	Yes
Treatment	Propranolol; surgery if symptoms are disabling	Propranolol; mitral valve replacement for severe mitral insufficiency

TABLE 13.2. *IHSS versus severe mitral regurgitation (MR)*

IHSS
1. EKG: LVH with strain common
   Chest films: cardiomegaly uncommon;
   therefore, electrocardiographic–radiologic
   discordance

MR
1. EKG: LVH with strain uncommon, but if present
   chest films will show cardiomegaly; therefore,
   electrocardiographic–radiologic concordance
2. More commonly, EKG: no LVH. Chest films:
   cardiomegaly; therefore, reverse electrocardiographic–radiologic discordance

effect of various postural and pharmacological maneuvers on the timing of the murmur in MVP separates it from the murmur of IHSS (Chap. 6).

Double apical impulse and brisk carotid pulses with midsystolic retraction can be noted in both entities. A prominent A wave, a fourth heart sound, and a sustained forceful apical impulse are more distinctive of IHSS. Left ventricular hypertrophy (LVH) by EKG is a frequent finding in IHSS except in its early latent forms, but is unusual in MVP even in the presence of significant mitral regurgitation (Table 13.2). In the differential diagnosis of a pansystolic murmur, comparison of electrocardiographic evidence of LVH and radiologic cardiomegaly are most helpful: In IHSS, LVH with a strain pattern is noted on the EKG but the chest films reveal no significant cardiomegaly except in the end stages and when heart failure has occurred, whereas in severe mitral regurgitation due to MVP or to rheumatic heart disease, the electrocardiogram often shows no LVH but the chest films show moderate to marked cardiomegaly. In severe mitral insufficiency due to MVP or to rheumatic heart disease, if the EKG should show LVH, the chest films would always display cardiomegaly (electrocardiographic–radiological concordance) whereas in IHSS with or without mitral regurgitation the EKG may show severe LVH in the absence of radiological cardiomegaly. There is, therefore, a frequent electrocardiographic–radiological discordance in IHSS (e.g., LVH by electrocardiography and no cardiomegaly on chest films but not in rheumatic or myxomatous mitral regurgitation in which LVH by EKG is never noted in the absence of marked cardiomegaly on chest films and in which a reverse discordance often occurs—marked radiological cardiomegaly associated with lack of electrocardiographic LVH). The explanation for these discordances lies in the volume overload and the associated left ventricular dilatation in mitral regurgitation as opposed to the pressure overload and left ventricular hypertrophy in IHSS. The echocardiographic features of the two conditions are distinctive (Table 13.1). In MVP there is an increased excursion of the anterior leaflet in early diastole with rapid posterior movement in mid-diastole whereas in IHSS a slow E-F slope due to decreased left ventricular compliance is not infrequent. In IHSS, systolic anterior motion (SAM) of the anterior leaflet is noted versus the posterior pansystolic or midsystolic motion of the leaflets in MVP. Angiographically, cavity obliteration with prominent papillary muscles, increased contractility, and abnormal position of the apex in the LAO and lateral views are common to both conditions. Since both MVP and IHSS can be associated with increased contractility, increased emptying of the left ventricle, and cavity obliteration (170), the diagnosis of IHSS should not be made merely on the basis of these findings. In IHSS, the anterior leaflet does not prolapse and outflow tract obstruction, due to anterior displacement of the edge of the anterior leaflet abutting against the hypertrophied septum, is observed; a V shaped filling defect due to this phenomenon is often noted on the posteroanterior left ventriculogram.

ASSOCIATION OF MVP WITH PRIMARY PULMONARY HYPERTENSION AND WITH PULMONARY EMPHYSEMA

MVP has been described in primary pulmonary hypertension (141) in an echocardiographic study of nine patients with this disorder. Four of the nine patients were found to have prolapse with angiographic confirmation in one and none had midsystolic click or late systolic murmur. To explain this association, the authors quoted studies indicating that primary pulmonary hypertension is a connective tissue disorder.

Salazar and Edwards (317) observed, on postmortem studies, an association of pulmonary emphysema and fibrosis in eight of their 37 cases of myxomatous valves. Conversely, the same group (150) has observed, in unselected material, "that among cases with pulmonary emphysema, some degree of myxomatous valvular change is not uncommon" and that, in these patients, the tricuspid valve, which is challenged by the associated right ventriculary hypertension, is more obviously involved. To explain the association of myxomatous mitral valve and pulmonary emphysema, a connective tissue disorder was postulated. Interestingly, Marfan's syndrome, a developmental disorder of connective tissue, is frequently associated with myxomatous MVP, and with a variety of pulmonary abnormalities including pulmonary emphysema (150) and air trapping.

While acknowledging the common association of myxomatous mitral valve and pulmonary emphysema in her necropsy material, Pomerance (279) has rightfully stated that "the importance of this association is difficult to assess in an urban hospital where chronic pulmonary pathology is a frequent finding."

Our group (400) studied pulmonary function in 20 nonsmokers with idiopathic MVP, of whom nine (45%) complained of dyspnea. The most common pulmonary function abnormalities were an increased residual volume (63% of patients studied) and a reduced steady state diffusing capacity

(50% of patients). There was no relationship between the presence of dyspnea with either the frequently encountered thoracic skeletal abnormalities, or the abnormality of pulmonary function. We postulated that the pulmonary function abnormalities reflect a pulmonary parenchymal disorder possibly secondary to a connective tissue disorder in the lung.

MVP AND MUSCULAR DYSTROPHY

MVP has been described in association with myotonic dystrophy (387) in one patient who had 25 relatives that were screened. Eight had evidence of both myotonic dystrophy and echocardiographic MVP and one had MVP alone. The propositus had a nonejection click followed by a late systolic murmur, but none of the relatives with MVP had any auscultatory abnormalities. Pathological studies in patients with myotonic dystrophy have shown the mitral valve to be normal.

The same group of workers (299) reported on echocardiographic screening in 29 other patients with myotonic dystrophy, and in 17 patients with Duchenne's muscular dystrophy. Five of the 29 patients (17%) with myotonic dystrophy and four of the 17 (23%) with Duchenne's dystrophy had MVP by echocardiography. In seven of the nine patients with abnormal echocardiograms, MVP was diagnosed by the finding of 3 mm pansystolic hammocking and in two by the finding of midsystolic dipping. Auscultatory findings were not reported in these patients. To the best of my knowledge, neither myxomatous degeneration of the mitral valve nor nonejection clicks [except in one case (387)] have been reported in muscular dystrophy. The association between MVP and muscular dystrophy could be coincidental and should be sought in other patients to determine if there is a chance association, a genetic linkage of two traits, or if MVP is secondary to a myopathy affecting the papillary muscle.

MVP AND ACROMEGALY

Systolic click and late systolic murmur were described in a patient with acromegaly (184). Myxomatous degeneration of the mitral valve has not been described in this disease. This case represents, probably, a random association of two entities.

SUMMARY

MVP is such a prevalent disorder that a chance association with other diseases should be expected. Extensive studies are needed to establish causal relationship or genetic linkage. Of all associations so far reported, only the association with connective tissue disorder (e.g., Marfan's syndrome and others) and with secundum atrial septal defect seem to be more prevalent than can be accounted for by chance.

Chapter 14

Prognosis and Complications

The prognosis for patients with MVP is generally favorable. However, the course of this syndrome may infrequently be complicated by progression of mitral insufficiency, with or without ruptured chordae tendineae, by bacterial endocarditis, malignant arrhythmias, and sudden death. These complications have shattered the illusion of innocence of this syndrome (368) which, "in some cases might be the harbinger of something much more sinister" (113). Yet, considering the prevalence of MVP and the relatively rare occurrence of complications, we must infer that this syndrome appears to have a generally benign course. Popp states, "Since there is probably a large pool of subclinical cases in the population, the overall prognosis would seem to be excellent" (283).

FOLLOW-UP STUDIES IN PATIENTS WITH MVP, DEVELOPMENT, AND PROGRESSION OF MITRAL INSUFFICIENCY

Several prospective and retrospective follow-up studies of idiopathic MVP have been published (5,8,26,28,201,253). The first such study was retrospective (5), and reported on 62 patients with isolated late systolic murmurs of whom 33 had a systolic click. These patients were followed for a minimum of 9 years (mean 13.8, maximum 22). In ten patients, there was slight deterioration marked, in most, by slight cardiac enlargement on X-ray films and by the development of pansystolic murmur in three. Of 62 patients, three died of irrelevant causes, one died from bacterial endocarditis and one died 11 years later at age 75 from increasing mitral insufficiency. One patient had chordal rupture that necessitated valve replacement and bacterial endocarditis caused heart failure in another patient. Altogether five patients developed bacterial endocarditis during their follow-up period. Of significance was the absence of deterioration in 41 patients over an average of 13.8 years, and the fact that sudden death did not occur.

Major deficiencies in this paper (which is often quoted as demonstrating a favorable prognosis in MVP) include (a) It is retrospective. (b) Patients with isolated clicks were excluded. Admittedly, their inclusion would have improved the overall prognosis since these patients have a better outlook than those with murmurs (253). (c) Patients with a history of chest pain or dyspnea were excluded. (d) Patients with an abnormal electrocardiogram were excluded because of the mistaken assumption that the ST-T changes in this syndrome are a manifestation of cardiomyopathy or coronary artery disease (19). (e) About one-half of these patients (29 of 62) had isolated late systolic murmur, a nonspecific finding frequently noted in mild rheumatic mitral insufficiency (175). As a matter of fact, 14 of the 62 patients gave a history of rheumatic fever. These cases dilute this follow-up study and detract from its value in the study of the long term prognosis of idiopathic MVP. None of these patients underwent echocardiographic or angiocardiographic studies that would have confirmed MVP.

This study reports, therefore, on a group of patients of whom one-half may have had mild rheumatic mitral insufficiency. In those with a click, the associated late systolic murmur would be expected to result in a relatively high incidence of bacterial endocarditis as shown in this study, but the exclusion of patients with ST-T wave abnormalities may have favorably altered the prognosis with reference to malignant arrhythmias and sudden death. Barlow and Pocock (19) rightfully stated that Allen et al.'s conclusion that "there is no justification for the belief that ventricular ectopics in their patients are dangerous" (5) would, therefore, seem to be rather tenuous. The interesting finding in this study is that only five patients, including one with endocarditis and one with ruptured chordae tendinea, have developed pansystolic murmur and significant mitral regurgitation.

Table 14.1 summarizes the data presented in the six available follow-up studies, including Allen et al.'s (5), which have reported on a total of 373 patients. Four of these studies are in abstract form and the data, therefore, is incomplete. The mean follow-up time was at least 4.2 years and some patients were followed for up to 40 years (8). One-half of these studies were retrospective and based on reevaluation of patients who had a midsystolic click or late systolic murmur (or both) documented phonocardiographically. Only one study (26) did not report on the auscultatory findings and was based purely on angiographic identification of MVP. Little information is available on the development of late systolic murmur in patients who had originally had isolated click. In only one study (201) this information is available with a late systolic murmur occurring on follow-up in four out of seven patients with isolated clicks. In a second study (8) which reported on 16 patients with isolated clicks (mean follow-up, 25 years) 12 patients developed multiple clicks or late systolic murmur but, unfortunately, no distinction is made between the two. More information is available on the development of pansystolic murmurs or severe mitral insufficiency in patients who originally had a click and/or late systolic murmurs [15% of the reported cases (35 out of 236) (Fig. 14.1)]. In at least four patients the pansystolic murmur resulted from endocarditis. It cannot be determined from these studies whether the development of mitral regurgitation was due to progression of the prolapse or to ruptured chordae tendineae. Ruptured chordae was documented in only 12 patients but it is possible that it may have been responsible for the development of mitral regurgitation in some of the re-

TABLE 14.1. Long term follow-up studies in MVP

	Allen et al. (5)	Bensman et al. (28)	Appelblatt et al. (8)	Belardi et al. (26)	Koch et al. (201)	Mills et al. (253)
Number of patients in whom information was available	62	14	69	137	38	53
Percentage of women	45%	NA	49%	NA	65%	64%
Mean age (years) when first seen	38	NA	NA	47.1	40.5	41.1
Follow-up time in years	13.8 Mean	4.2 Mean	10–40	4.2 Mean	> 10	13.7 Mean
Prospective (P) Retrospective (R)	R	P	R	P	P	R
Development of late systolic murmur in patients with isolated click	NA	NA	12/16 (1)	NA	4/7	NA
Basis for diagnosis of MVP	Auscultation	Auscultation and echocardiography	Auscultation	Angiography	Auscultation	Auscultation
Development of pansystolic murmur or severe mitral regurgitation in patients with click and/or late systolic murmur	9/16 (2)	3/14	11/69	NA (3)	6/38	7/53 (4)
Ruptured chordae tendineae	2	1	None	7	NA	2
Infective endocarditis	5	None	None	3	None	3
Sudden death	None	None	1	2	5	1 (Quinidine) 1 Ventricular fibrillation successfully resuscitated

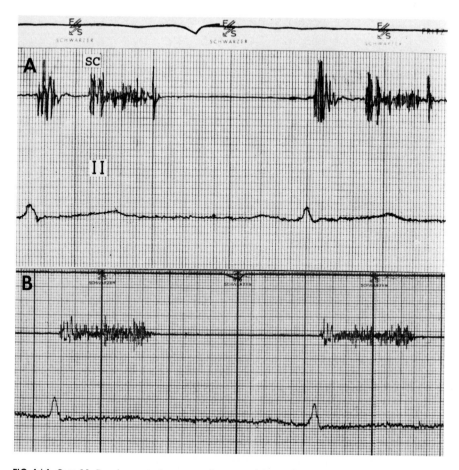

FIG. 14.1. *Case 11.* Development of a pansystolic murmur **(B)** in a 61-year-old man who, 4 years earlier, had midsystolic clicks (sc) followed by a late systolic murmur **(A)**.

maining patients. Infective endocarditis occurred in 11 patients out of 373 that were followed. Sudden death and/or successfully resuscitated ventricular fibrillation (one patient) occurred in 10 of the 373 patients (2.7%). In these follow up studies, complications were more frequent in men than in women (8,253).

The main points presented by each of the six studies require further comments. Bensman et al. (28) eliminated four of their 18 patients, two with late systolic murmur and two with isolated clicks, because of a normal echocardiogram. The elimination of two patients with late systolic murmur is warranted but that of the isolated click patients is not, because false-negative echocardiograms are not infrequent. The mean follow-up period in this study is brief (4 years). In the same study, three patients with late systolic murmurs and midsystolic click on the initial examination demonstrated progression to a pansystolic murmur, and two of the three developed heart failure requiring mitral valve surgery. In one of the two cases, ruptured chordae tendineae was noted but in the other mitral regurgitation was due to progression of the MVP with markedly dilated mitral valve annulus. In most cases, auscultatory findings and clinical state remained unchanged over a relatively short follow-up time.

Appelblatt et al.'s (8) study is retrospective and has the advantage of a long follow-up time of 10 to 40 years in 69 patients. Fifteen of these patients died and, according to life expectancy tables, fourteen would have died at time of follow-up. The average age at death was 68 years, a reassuring finding, and survival was not less than expected. The authors noted that men more often than women had progression of auscultatory findings and that sudden cardiac death was rare (one patient).

Belardi et al. (26) reported on the largest group of patients so far studied, but the follow-up time was short (mean 4.2 years) and the diagnosis of MVP was made by angiocardiography alone with no report on auscultatory or echocardiographic data. The authors rightly excluded MVP due to coronary artery disease. Mitral valve replacement was performed in 11 patients for severe mitral regurgitation (ruptured chordae tendineae in seven). This finding merely indicates that "floppy" mitral valve is a common cause of severe mitral regurgitation, and does not provide us with information on the development and progression of mitral regurgitation in a group of patients who have a click with or without a late systolic murmur or who have a positive echocardiogram with or without auscultatory findings. Two of their patients died suddenly (neither had significant mitral regurgitation at the time of the study), and three developed bacterial endocarditis. Three of their patients developed complete heart block requiring permanent pacemakers. Most of these complications occurred in patients with mitral regurgitation on the initial study, and the authors concluded that "the majority of patients with idiopathic MVP have a benign course."

The ten year prospective follow-up study of Koch et al. (201) provides information on all patients initially reported by this group (154) in 1966. The major finding in this study was a relatively high incidence of sudden death (five patients aged nine, 30,32,50, and 64 years respectively, with no evidence of coronary artery disease). In this study, echocardiography was diagnostic of MVP in 15 out of 22 patients (68%) with known auscultatory findings. There was a higher prevalence of positive echocardiograms in those patients who had a late systolic murmur in addition to the click (15 of 18 or 83%). None of these patients required mitral valve surgery. The authors concluded that "while this group contained a high proportion with symptoms, obvious auscultatory and electrocardiographic changes and thus may not represent the whole population with this condition, these results suggest a less favorable natural history in many instances than is usually considered to be the case."

The excellent study of Mills et al. (253), although retrospective, provides very helpful information on the long term prognosis of idiopathic MVP (see Table 14.1). The authors, who examined the natural history of this syndrome in 53 patients, unfortunately included isolated late systolic murmur, a nonspecific auscultatory finding, in their series (18 out of 53 patients). The remainder of their patients had either isolated clicks (22 patients) or click and late systolic murmur (13 patients). The authors compensated for this inclusion, which detracts from the value of the study, by performing echocardiography on 36 of the 53 patients. The echocardiogram was diagnostic of MVP in 33 and negative in three who had isolated clicks. Breakdown of auscultatory findings in patients with positive echocardiograms was not reported, but I have to assume that some of the 18 patients with isolated late systolic murmurs had positive echocardiograms that warrants, therefore, their inclusion in a study on MVP. To preclude bias in patient selection, phonocardiographic records were used as the only source in selecting the population to be studied. Nine patients died during the follow-up, but in only two was death related to the MVP. One of these patients had bacterial endocarditis and chordal rupture, and sudden death occurred in another patient with severe mitral regurgitation who was on quinidine. There were six other major complications related to the MVP. One patient developed ventricular fibrillation that was successfully resuscitated, two developed bacterial endocarditis, and three severe mitral regurgitation with ruptured chordae in one. The remaining 38 patients were alive and well on follow-up evaluation with minor symptoms of chest pain, palpitations, and dyspnea essentially unchanged. In analyzing the prognostic factors, the authors found that the complications that occurred in a total of eight patients (15%) "were significantly ($p = 0.15$) associated with a late systolic murmur rather than an isolated midsystolic click." Complications were more common in men and older patients but this finding was not statistically significant. On the basis of these data, the authors felt that the diagnosis of MVP should not be regarded as ominous; however, patients in whom this diagnosis is associated with a late systolic murmur should be followed carefully because severe complications may occur.

It is not possible to explain the contradictory prognostic information provided by these six studies. These contrasting results may be due to the different selection factors in the population studied (253). For instance, the favorable outlook in Allen et al.'s series (5) may be explained by the exclusion of patients with abnormal EKGs and abnormal X-ray films and the inclusion of patients with late systolic murmur due to insignificant rheumatic mitral regurgitation. On the other hand, the poor outlook reported by Koch et al. (201) may be explained by the high prevalence of abnormal EKGs in their patients (36 out of 40). I believe that the selection process provides only a partial explanation for these discrepancies and that further prospective studies are needed to provide us with definite information on the long term prognosis of this prevalent syndrome. It should be realized that prognostic studies have been reported on patients seen in cardiology services and do not provide follow-up information on the asymptomatic patient in whom MVP is detected on a routine physical examination or by echocardiography during an epidemiological survey. It is not unreasonable to assume that the prognosis in this group of subjects will be found to be more favorable than the former group. I am not aware of any follow-up study in patients with "silent" MVP. We are planning such a study on a group of patients, first diagnosed as having "silent" MVP at least 4 years ago.

In summary, the long term prognosis in idiopathic MVP is benign and favorable despite the rare occurrence of major complications. Patients with mitral insufficiency as evidenced by late systolic or pansystolic murmurs are probably at a higher risk for these complications and deserve careful watching and more aggressive management. The presence of a late systolic murmur may be an indication that these patients belong to a subset prone to progression of prolapse and the resulting mitral insufficiency may offer favorable conditions for the development of endocarditis.

In the absence of ruptured chordae tendineae and endocarditis the development and progression of mitral insufficiency is probably a rare event in patients initially seen with "silent" MVP, isolated clicks, or clicks with late systolic murmur. I concur with Barlow and Pocock's assessment of the risk of development of progressive mitral insufficiency in this syndrome (19): "It would seem to us impossible to predict in any individual case whether progression to pure severe mitral regurgitation will occur, but in the absence of infective endocarditis it is probable that the majority of patients deteriorate only slightly, or not at all over many years," but I would modify this statement by adding "in the absence of ruptured chordae tendineae."

The natural history of "floppy" mitral valve, an advanced form of MVP, is still unknown. It is possible that these patients may have displayed only echocardiographic or phonocardiographic evidence of MVP initially with subsequent appearance, in succession, of click, late systolic, and then pansystolic murmurs (175,306,307,336) (Table 3.1). However, progression of these findings in a large group of patients has not been documented yet. Most patients with "floppy" mitral valves and severe mitral insufficiency are referred with the diagnosis of rheumatic mitral regurgitation and MVP is detected by echocardiography, left ventricular angiography, surgical exploration, or at necropsy. In a significant percentage, associated chordal rupture is noted. In a large majority of these patients a previous history of a click with or without a late systolic murmur cannot be obtained. Most of these patients are in their fifties or sixties and a click, if it were present at an earlier age, may have been missed because of lack of appreciation of this auscultatory finding before the late 1960s. Moreover, echocardiography was not available then to shed some light on the natural history of "floppy" mitral valve and the possible gradual development of mitral regurgitation in patients with idiopathic MVP.

The long term prognosis of MVP and the natural history of this syndrome and of its advanced form, the "floppy" mitral valve, offer a fertile field for future investigations. Future follow-up studies should not include late systolic murmur unless echocardiographic or angiographic confirmation of prolapse is obtained.

RUPTURED CHORDAE TENDINEAE

The natural history of idiopathic MVP may be suddenly interrupted by the occurrence of a cardiac catastrophe—ruptured chordae tendineae (Figs. 14.2A to 14.6). This complication may result in overwhelming mitral insufficiency or in sudden worsening of mitral regurgitation followed by hemodynamic adjustment and clinical stabilization with subsequent gradual deterioration. Many workers presented evidence implicating myxomatous transformation of the mitral valve and the resulting MVP as a major and common cause of ruptured chordae tendineae (5,14,26,28,57,77,142,150, 157,213,229,237,244,253,278,292,293,319,330,336,338,339,396). More than 125 cases of ruptured chordae tendineae in association with proven myxomatous MVP (necropsy or surgery) are included in these reports. In my series, ruptured chordae tendineae was confirmed at surgery in five patients with myxomatous mitral valve and severe mitral regurgitation. Chordal rupture in MVP may be secondary to infective endocarditis (5,213, 253,293), but in most reported cases no history of previous endocarditis could be elicited (14).

The first report of ruptured chordae tendineae of a myxomatous mitral valve appeared in 1966 (237). Six patients were described with ruptured chordae, "voluminous supple leaflets, dilatation of the mitral annulus, and absence of fibrotic or inflammatory changes in the chordae." Every one of these patients had known of the existence of a heart murmur for years before the development of serious heart symptoms. The authors did not report microscopic findings and did not recognize the myxomatous transformation, but their description of the voluminous leaflets and large annulus is characteristic of myxomatous MVP. The largest number of chordal rupture of a myxomatous valve has been reported in three series that have stressed the importance of "floppy" mitral valve as a major cause of pure mitral insufficiency. In one series of 50 patients with "floppy" mitral valve (77), 19 patients (38%) were found to have ruptured chordae tendineae at surgery; in a second series (319) of 66 patients with "floppy" mitral valve 41 (62%) had ruptured chordae tendineae at surgery, and in a third series (244) 31 of 38 patients with "floppy" mitral valve who underwent mitral valve replacement had chordal rupture (82%). Ruptured chordae tendineae may

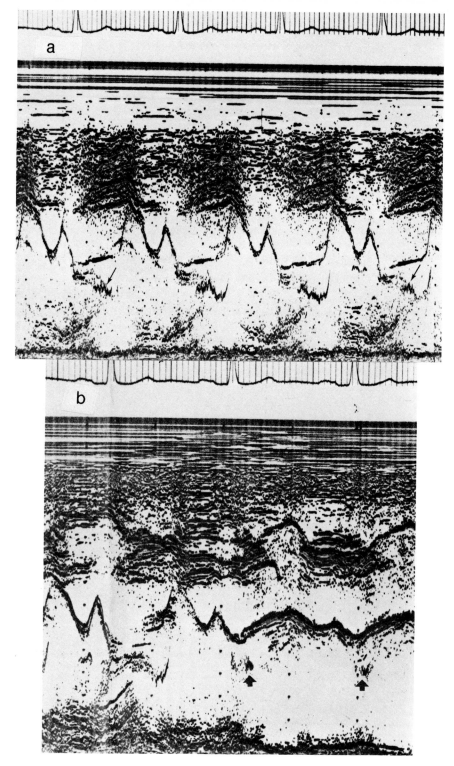

FIG. 14.2A. *Case 210.* Echocardiogram in surgically proven ruptured chordae to a myxomatous posterior leaflet, in a 46-year-old man. **a.** Late systolic dipping and moderately high frequency systolic fluttering of the posterior leaflet (*arrow*). **b.** Linear systolic echoes (*arrows*) within the normally echo-free left atrium. Note beginning of paradoxical anterior motion of posterior leaflet during diastole (**a** and **b**).

occur in patients with MVP and symptomatic severe mitral regurgitation leading to acute exacerbation of symptoms or in patients with minimal myxomatous changes of the valve and minimal symptoms leading to acute mitral insufficiency (77,157). Therefore, sudden deterioration in a patient with known mitral regurgitation and "floppy" mitral valve or the sudden occurrence of severe mitral regurgitation are often due to ruptured chordae tendineae; 17 of 20 patients with acute onset of symptoms had chordal rupture at the time of operation in one series (319). However, a history of dramatic onset of symptoms or sudden deterioration may not be present (319) and ruptured chordae are noted either on echocardiography or at surgery.

The sudden development of ruptured chordae tendineae in patients with known nonejection click and late systolic murmur has been documented in a few patients (28,142,253). One of these patients (142) was seen 6 years earlier because of chest pain, palpitations, a loud click, and a Grade II/VI late systolic murmur; 6 years later at age 58, she developed severe

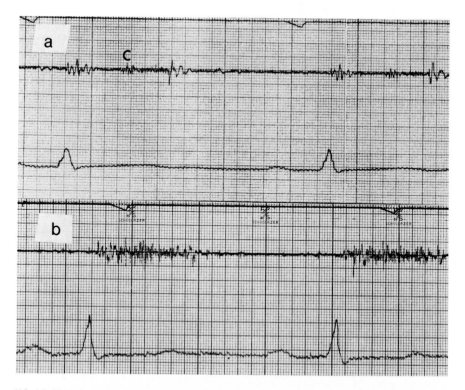

FIG. 14. 2B. Case 18. Phonocardiograms (a and b) recorded 4 years apart in a 46-year-old man with probable ruptured chordae tendineae. The first phonocardiogram (a) shows a midsystolic click (c) followed by a late systolic murmur. (See Fig. 12.11 for left cineventriculogram). The second phonocardiogram (b) was taken following the sudden onset of severe left ventricular failure. Note isolated pansystolic murmur.

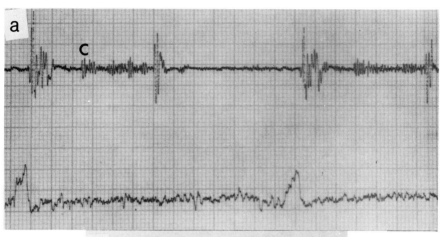

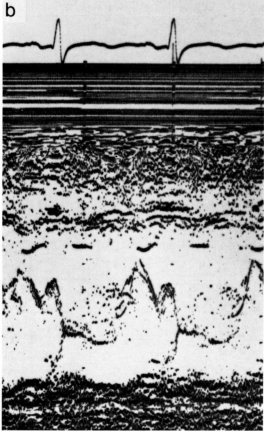

FIG. 14.3. *Case 74.* 51-year-old man who developed probable chordal rupture in 1977. Phonocardiogram (a) had shown a midsystolic click (c) followed by a late systolic murmur (1971). Echocardiogram (b) had shown a midsystolic dipping (1973). (See Figs. 14.4 and 14.8 for further details).

heart failure and a pansystolic murmur and required urgent surgery. I encountered sudden deterioration associated with the development of a pansystolic murmur and followed by relative stabilization in two patients known to have had a midsystolic click and a late systolic murmur. I suspect ruptured chordae tendineae in these patients who are scheduled for mitral valve replacement (Figs. 14.2B,14.3,14.4, and 14.8). Harvey (264) reported a case of a 45-year-old physician with known isolated click for 25 years who developed, 4 years ago, a Grade IV holosystolic murmur, progressive cardiomegaly, and evidence of cardiac decompensation. Echocardiography and left ventriculography demonstrated MVP. Chordal rupture is postulated but has not been confirmed in this patient in whom mitral valve replacement is planned.

I am not aware of any published case with isolated midsystolic click and, therefore, no mitral regurgitation or of any case of "silent" MVP in whom subsequent chordal rupture was documented. This may indicate that the superimposed mitral regurgitation may be a contributing factor in the chordal rupture or that the occurrence of a murmur of mitral regurgitation may indicate a progressive form of MVP prone to the development of chordal rupture. The absence of reported rupture in isolated midsystolic click adds a further argument to Mills et al.'s (253) contention that patients with isolated clicks have a favorable prognosis with rare major complications.

In MVP, the chordae attached to the posterior leaflet are more commonly ruptured than the anterior leaflet chordae (157,292,338) but rupture of the latter has also been reported (396). The more common involvement of the posterior leaflet by the myxomatous process may explain the greater frequency of rupture of the posterior cusp chordae. Of the chordae attached to the three scallops of the posterior leaflet, those attached to the middle scallop have the higher tendency to rupture. Anterior chordal rupture may occur more frequently than several surgical series would suggest, but it may be more catastrophic and is, therefore, seen in coroners' autopsies (157).

In follow-up studies in MVP, ruptured chordae tendineae was infrequent (Table 14.1) and occurred in only five patients out of 226 followed, excluding the seven cases of Bellardi et al. (26) who had their rupture prior to their inclusion in this angiographic series. In their study on the association of secundum atrial septal defect with MVP Leachman et al. (213) reported on three patients with intact chordae on the first operation with

---

→

FIG. 14.4. *Case 74.* Phonocardiogram, echocardiogram, and left ventriculogram in a 51-year-old man who developed sudden heart failure associated with a pansystolic murmur. Chordal rupture is felt likely. a. Phonocardiogram shows pansystolic murmur. b. Echocardiogram shows coarse diastolic fluttering of the posterior leaflet (arrow) with paradoxical anterior movement of this leaflet. Note heavy diastolic echoes behind posterior leaflet and shaggy echoes behind anterior leaflet. c. Echocardiogram shows late systolic buckling of posterior leaflet. d. Left cineventriculogram (LAO) shows MVP with moderately severe to severe mitral regurgitation. Arrow points to prolapsing posterior leaflet. (See Figs. 14.3 and 14.8).

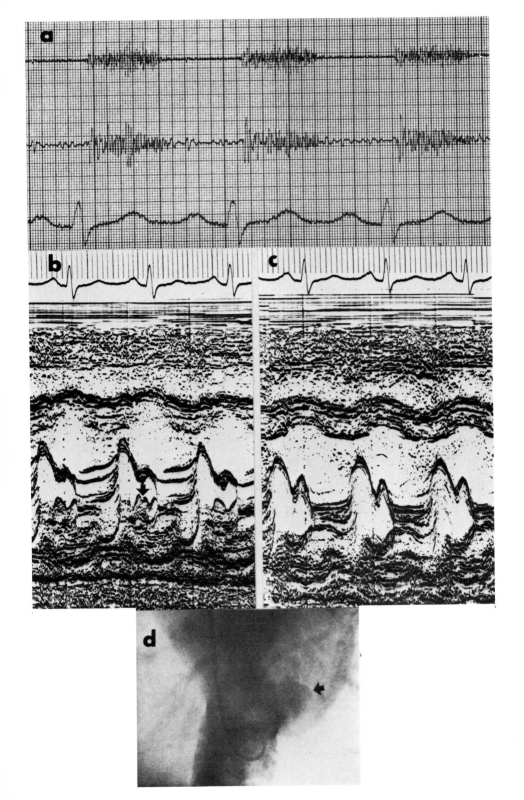

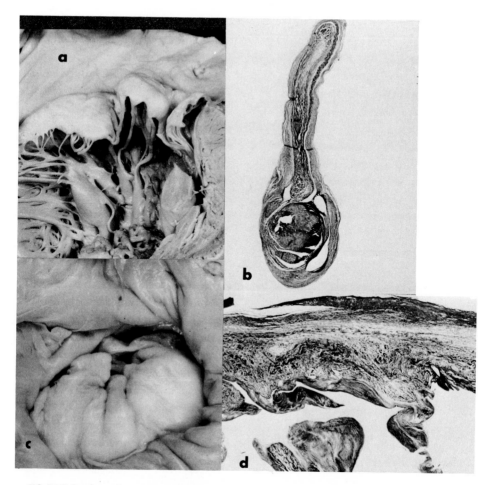

FIG. 14.5. Specimens from a 59-year-old man with spontaneous rupture of mitral chordae. a. A portion of the mitral valve. The segment to which chordae have ruptured shows prolapse of greater degree than is evident in the related segments of the valve, which also show some degree of prolapse. b. Low power photomicrograph of the ruptured end of a cord. Elastic tissue stain; ×12. c. The unopened mitral valve viewed from above. There is widespread hooding of the leaflets toward the left antrium. d. Photomicrograph of nonruptured segment of the posterior mitral leaflet showing characteristic features of myxomatous change along with secondary fibrous thickening on each aspect of the leaflet. Elastic tissue stain; ×13. (Courtesy of Drs. Richard B. Guthrie and Jesse E. Edwards. From ref. 150. By permission)

subsequent rupture requiring mitral valve replacement 2, 6, and 6 years later respectively. Three of these patients had mitral regurgitation on the initial operation and auscultatory findings were not reported.

Pathologically, the chordae in MVP are delicate and long, but may be short and thickened (150). The abnormally increased length of the chordae may be the result of myxomatous transformation of these structures. However, "though such changes have been observed, they are nevertheless un-

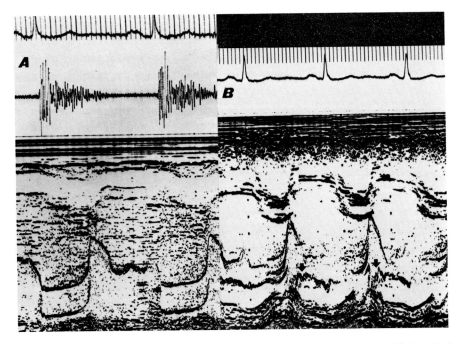

FIG. 14.6. Phonocardiogram and echocardiogram in a 50-year-old man who developed, suddenly, a loud pansystolic murmur, presumably due to ruptured chordae tendineae. A. Phonocardiogram shows a pansystolic murmur and echocardiogram a pansystolic sagging. B. Echocardiogram shows coarse diastolic fluttering of the posterior leaflet (arrows).

common, leaving the probability that the major cause of increased chordal length is a consequence of abnormal tension upon these structures by the leaflets prolapsing toward the left atrium" (150). This increased tension may lead to lengthening, thinning, and rupture (339).

Current evidence indicates that myxomatous transformation of the mitral valve is probably the commonest cause of "spontaneous" chordal rupture (150,279,336). This evidence is based on the site of chordal rupture to the posterior leaflet, the leaflet most commonly involved in prolapse (157,338). The prior documentation of midsystolic click and late systolic murmur in a few patients prior to chordal rupture constitutes another circumstantial evidence (28,142,253). However, the most convincing evidence comes from the demonstration both grossly and histologically of myxomatous involvement of elements of the valve not involved in chordal rupture (150,336) (Fig. 14.5). Moreover, friction lesions of the left ventricular endocardium commonly noted in idiopathic MVP (278,317) have been observed in relation to the chordae that have ruptured (278,336). In a few reported cases of chordal rupture, myxomatous transformation of the chordae has been noted (57,244,396). In one series (244), for instance, which reported a high frequency of ruptured chordae confirmed at surgery (31 out of 38), the

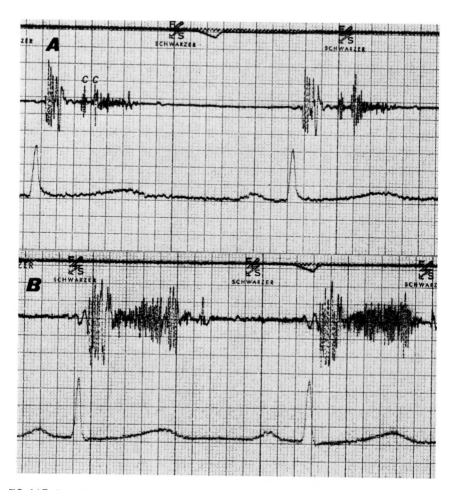

FIG. 14.7. *Case 57.* Endocarditis and MVP in a 50-year-old man who had clicks (c) and a late systolic murmur on admission to the hospital (A). During hospitalization, he developed a pansystolic murmur (B).

chordae were described as having varying degrees of disorganization of the collagen core and "circumferential deposition of myxomatous tissue."

Ruptured chordae tendineae in idiopathic MVP should be suspected whenever rapid deterioration and progression of symptoms occurs. The sudden development of a pansystolic murmur or a midsystolic murmur radiating to the base of the heart provides additional confirmatory evidence. Echocardiography reveals a flail anterior or posterior leaflet (123). Coarse, irregular, anterior diastolic motion of the posterior leaflet is noted and is probably due to a Venturi effect created by diastolic flow from the left atrium to the left ventricle, drawing anteriorly the flail posterior leaflet (160) (Figs. 14.4 and 14.6). However, abnormal paradoxical motion per se may be observed in "floppy" mitral valve with intact chordae tendineae (255) (Fig. 9.14).

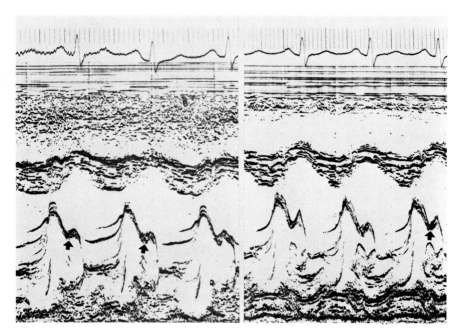

FIG. 14.8. *Case 74.* Shaggy echoes (*arrows*) behind the anterior leaflet in a 51-year-old man with idiopathic MVP, presumed ruptured chordae and no history of endocarditis. Note coarse diastolic fluttering of posterior leaflet. (See Figs. 14.3 and 14.4 for further details).

Feigenbaum states, "For all practical purpose, a severely prolapsing mitral valve and a flail valve may be functionally identical" (123). When the anterior leaflet is flail, the usual finding is marked irregularity of its motion in diastole (99,123). Pansystolic sagging of the mitral leaflets can be seen in ruptured chordae tendineae and flail leaflets, regardless of the etiology of the rupture and does not help, therefore, identify underlying myxomatous transformation (80,99,280). In the absence of chaotic diastolic vibrations of a mitral leaflet it is difficult to differentiate MVP from ruptured chordae (280). Fine systolic fluttering of the mitral leaflet was described recently in five patients with ruptured chordae tendineae (251) and was ascribed to the action of high velocity blood flow upon the leaflet margin that has lost its support. I encountered this finding in two of my patients with MVP and ruptured chordae (Fig. 14.2A). Systolic left atrial echoes have also been observed (160) (Fig. 14.2A) and may originate from either a flail anterior or posterior mitral leaflet; however, they can be observed in MVP in the absence of chordal rupture. Midsystolic buckling of the mitral leaflets is not seen when ruptured chordae is superimposed on a prolapsed leaflet (101). Visualization of the freely mobile chordae has been noted but is rare (108).

Left ventricular angiography reveals the characteristic findings of MVP (Fig. 14.4) but significant mitral regurgitation may prevent adequate visu-

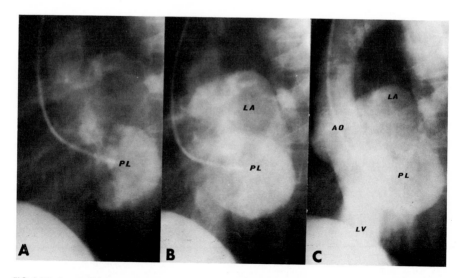

FIG. 14.9. *Case 3.* LV angiogram in the LAO projection showing prolapse of posterior leaflet (PL) into left atrium (LA): "Ballon sign." Three sequences (A, B, and C). Moderate MR. Patient died suddenly. (From ref. 171. By permission)

alization of the valve. The marked billowing of the leaflets and their wide excursion may be suggestive of chordal rupture, but the left ventriculogram does not often differentiate massive isolated MVP from chordal rupture.

In summary, ruptured chordae tendineae is a relatively rare complication of idiopathic MVP, a prevalent entity. However, MVP is probably the most common cause of primary or idiopathic ruptured chordae tendineae, a relatively rare mitral disorder.

INFECTIVE ENDOCARDITIS

Infective endocarditis is a major, but relatively infrequent, complication of idiopathic MVP. Several series and case reports have documented its occurrence in about 110 patients with MVP (5,13,26,55,75,80,108,156,157,184, 196,208,210,213,225,229,244,253,264,269,277,278,281,293,297,313,328, 334,339,346,348,373). Five of my 350 patients developed endocarditis (Fig. 14.7). The first report of bacterial endocarditis complicating MVP was published in 1964 by Facquet et al. (120).

The pathologic basis for endocarditis in MVP is considered by some workers (336) to be "trauma to the contact aspect of prolapsing segments as they make faulty contact with opposite elements of the valve during ventricular systole." Others (278,279) described areas of endocardial ulceration resulting from stretching of the cusp and the overlying endocardium as a site of endocarditis. The loss of endocardial continuity would invite the deposition of fibrin (278). A rare focus of endocarditis is the mural endocardium at sites of friction by chordae of the prolapsing leaflet (208). In this case report, the mitral cusps that were not involved by endocarditis were described as normal but the published illustration showed marked hooding consistent with myxomatous degeneration.

Prevalence of Endocarditis in Idiopathic MVP

Considering the prevalence of idiopathic MVP in the general population, infective endocarditis, which has been reported in 115 patients with this syndrome, is a relatively rare complication. In follow-up studies (5,8,26,28, 201,253) covering 373 patients (Table 14.1) with a mean follow-up time of four to 20 years, only 11 cases of endocarditis were reported. The largest number of this complication (5 cases) was reported in one series (5) which included, probably, a high prevalence of rheumatic heart disease manifested by isolated late systolic murmur. Likewise, in other series and other case reports, late systolic murmur was accepted as the sole evidence of MVP. It is possible, therefore, that some of the 120 patients reported as having MVP and endocarditis may have had underlying rheumatic heart disease. Although endocarditis is a relatively rare complication of MVP, MVP is frequently found as the underlying disorder in patients with endocarditis and particularly in those with mitral regurgitation. For example, of 87 consecutive patients diagnosed as having infective endocarditis at Stanford University Medical Center, ten (11%) had MVP and these 10 patients constituted more than one-third of the total group of 28 patients who had endocarditis associated with mitral regurgitation (80).

In most reports (5,80,278) there was a male preponderance. Although Lachman et al. (210) found that only four of their 10 patients were male, they have reported only on patients who had nonejection clicks and late systolic murmur and have therefore excluded patients with MVP and pansystolic murmur. The exclusion of patients with pansystolic murmur who are predominantly male would account for the female proponderance in this series.

Underlying Auscultatory Findings in Endocarditis Associated with MVP

To the best of my knowledge, occurrence of infective endocarditis in "silent" MVP has not been documented except possibly in one case, a 47-year-old woman admitted in 1973 with a pansystolic murmur and endocarditis due to streptococcal viridans and in whom no murmur was noted on physical examination carried out 5 years earlier (269). It is possible that a nonejection click may have been missed in 1968 since little attention was paid to this auscultatory finding at that time. Only a few cases of bacterial endocarditis occurring in patients with isolated nonejection clicks have been reported. The first such case was reported by LeBauer et al. (216); streptococcal viridans endocarditis had occurred 6 weeks after dental cleaning and resulted in transient late systolic murmur during the acute illness. Three other cases mentioned by Harvey (in ref. 264) probably included LeBauer et al.'s case which was reported from the same institution. In one of Harvey's cases (264) ruptured chordae tendineae with severe mitral regurgitation resulted from endocarditis. Another case of endocarditis was reported by Kincaid et al. (196). It occurred in an eight-year-old girl with isolated click; a late systolic murmur developed in the course of the endocarditis and could be elicited only with isometric exercise on follow-up visits. To these cases should be added two other reported by Lachman et al. (210) (patients were 11 and 15 years of age respectively) for a total of six to seven cases of endocarditis occurring in patients with isolated clicks. Of interest is the development of endocarditis in three of these patients a few weeks to a few months after dental cleaning (196,216) or dental therapy (210).

The great majority of patients with endocarditis and MVP either give a history of midsystolic click and late systolic murmur or of a pansystolic murmur heard on a previous examination or exhibit these auscultatory findings when they are first seen with the clinical picture of endocarditis (5,80, 210,253).

The above findings do not necessarily indicate that patients with "silent" MVP or with isolated midsystolic click are not at risk of developing endocarditis. The late systolic or pansystolic murmur, which is heard during the acute illness, may be due to the damage inflicted by the endocarditis on the myxomatous valve and the resulting mitral insufficiency. Of the 25 patients reported by one group (80) only 17 had a history of a previous heart murmur before the appearance of the endocarditis, and the other eight may have had clicks, late systolic or pansystolic murmur, or none of these auscultatory findings. In another series of ten patients with MVP and endocarditis (210), "the mitral valve abnormality was diagnosed for the first time during the current illness" in seven patients.

The late systolic murmur in MVP may become pansystolic in the course of endocarditis (80,334) indicating further damage to the mitral valve and possibly ruptured chordae tendineae, leaflet perforation, and so forth. A previously heard click associated with late systolic murmur may not be audible during the acute episode (80).

Recognition of MVP in Patients with Endocarditis

In patients with unexplained fever and insidious vague symptoms, the recognition of underlying MVP would raise the probability of endocarditis. A nonejection click and a soft late systolic murmur should be diligently sought by carefully listening to the patient in the supine, left lateral, standing, and even squatting positions. Late systolic accentuation of pansystolic murmur and T wave inversion in the inferior leads should raise the index of suspicion of MVP in patients with suspected or confirmed endocarditis (80). The high prevalence of pansystolic murmur during endocarditis complicating MVP makes the recognition of MVP difficult. In the presence of endocarditis, the echocardiographic diagnosis of MVP is valid because endocarditis per se does not cause the valve to prolapse as a consequence of infection. A late systolic dipping in such patients can be considered as specific of MVP. However, a pansystolic sagging can be encountered not only in idiopathic MVP but also in ruptured chordae tendineae resulting from endocarditis and cannot be used, therefore, as a means to identify MVP.

The usefulness of echocardiography in patients with suspected endocarditis and patients with positive blood cultures and normal auscultatory findings has not been established yet. It is possible that echocardiography in a few patients may unmask "silent" MVP pointing, therefore, to endocarditis. However, as mentioned above, the occurrence of endocarditis in previously or persistently "silent" MVP has not been reported yet.

In patients with known MVP, echocardiography can be helpful in the diagnosis of superimposed endocarditis by showing thickened, shaggy echoes suggestive of mitral valvular vegetation (80). In one series, however, (373) vegetations could not be demonstrated by echocardiography in 13 patients with MVP and endocarditis. It should also be kept in mind that the same shaggy echoes were described in patients with MVP in the absence of clinical evidence of endocarditis (61,373) and were ascribed to leaflet thickening and redundancy (Figs. 9.3,14.4, and 14.8).

Bacteriology of Endocarditis Complicating MVP

The spectrum of organisms seen in these patients is similar to that reported in other types of heart disease with predominance of alpha streptococcal infection (80,175). However, one group (210) has reported a high prevalence of streptococcus albus infection (six out of ten patients) noting that in their hospital this organism was often responsible for endocarditis especially in subjects who are on long term penicillin prophylaxis against rheumatic activity.

Prognostic Implications

The prevalence of pansystolic murmurs in patients with MVP and active endocarditis or with a previous history of endocarditis (80,244) "may reflect the deterioration in mitral valve function associated with infection" (80). Many of these patients are subsequently shown to have ruptured chordae tendineae (80,244). The development of a late systolic murmur in patients with isolated clicks, and of a pansystolic murmur in patients with previously documented late systolic murmur are further indications of mitral valve deterioration. It is possible, however, that the high prevalence of pansystolic murmurs in patients with MVP and bacterial endocarditis may indicate an increased susceptibility to endocarditis in patients with MVP and more severe regurgitation.

In patients with MVP, endocarditis, and ruptured chordae tendineae, the development of heart failure during the acute episode would indicate that the rupture resulted from the infection (80). However, in another group of patients, the chordal rupture may have antedated the infection and may have increased susceptibility to endocarditis because of the development or worsening of mitral regurgitation. In one series (80), nine out of 25 patients underwent mitral valve replacement after the episode of endocarditis and six were found to have ruptured chordae but the relationship of chordal rupture to the acute episode is not evident.

A few deaths resulting from endocarditis in MVP have been reported (5,80). Mitral valve aneurysm after infective endocarditis in MVP was reported (277). The patient underwent mitral valve replacement 9 years after the infectious episode. Two large perforations of a voluminous anterior leaflet were noted.

Indications for Antibiotics Prophylaxis in MVP

Documentation of endocarditis in MVP has lead many workers to recommend antibiotic prophylaxis against infective endocarditis in all patients with MVP regardless of their physical findings (196,210,264,269). In a recently published statement prepared by the Committee on Rheumatic Fever and Bacterial Endocarditis of the Council on Cardiovascular Disease in the Young of American Heart Association (Prevention of Bacterial Endocarditis) (401) prophylaxis is recommended in patients with MVP syndrome with mitral insufficiency. In a footnote it is stated that "although cases of infective endocarditis in mitral valve prolapse syndrome have been documented the incidence appears to be relatively low and the necessity of prophylaxis in all of these patients has not yet been established" (401). Others (348), having noted that the majority of their patients "had their teeth extracted without development of bacterial endocarditis," felt that "prophylaxis may not be necessary." Shortly thereafter (346) they modified their recommendations after they encountered endocarditis in a young man with a nonejection click and a late systolic murmur.

The following available data already reviewed should be taken into consideration in formulating a rational policy on antibiotic prophylaxis in MVP. (a) Endocarditis is a rare complication in a prevalent syndrome which is frequently encountered in young healthy individuals and which may be present in almost 4% of the general population. Only 115 cases of this association have been reported. Endocarditis is a rare complication in long term follow-up studies of MVP and some of the reported cases of endocarditis may have occurred in patients with rheumatic mitral regurgitation rather than in patients with MVP. In a study of 74 women with MVP among 1,169 surveyed (286), none had endocarditis despite lack of prophylaxis and "in spite of a myriad of potential incidence of bacteremia, parturition, dental manipulation, and elective operations." (b) Endocarditis has not been reported in "silent" MVP. (c) Only six cases of endocarditis associated with isolated clicks have been reported. (d) The great majority of patients with MVP who have developed endocarditis had a cardiac murmur, either late systolic or pansystolic in duration. We should keep in mind that the murmur in MVP may be evanescent or only induced by various maneuvers. The significance of transient or provoked murmur has not been established yet. However, the detection of this murmur in patients presenting with endocarditis may be a manifestation of valve damage by the infection in patients who may have had isolated clicks or a silent form of MVP. Only prospective studies of these two groups of patients would establish the risk of developing SBE.

On the basis of the above data, my current policy, which has to be flexible because of conflicting information and which may be modified in the future as further prospective studies are reported, is as follows: (a) I do not recommend endocarditis prophylaxis in "silent" MVP provided no murmur can be elicited in various positions including squatting. (b) I recommend prophylaxis according to the American Heart Association's recent antibiotic schedule (401) in patients with MVP and late or pansystolic murmur (80,253). (c) In patients with isolated click and no murmur induced by various maneuvers, I do not recommend antibiotic prophylaxis for dental cleaning, dental extraction, and surgical interventions in the absence of infection. However, I recommend prophylaxis in dental procedures or surgical interventions that are to be carried out on an infected site or focus.

In formulating these recommendations, I am mindful of the side effects and complications of various antibiotics used for prophylaxis. The risk of an adverse reaction to antibiotics outweighs the benefit to be derived in patients at very low risk of developing endocarditis.

Some workers (12) who have shown angiographic MVP in patients with coronary artery disease have recommended antibiotic prophylaxis in this setting, in the absence of auscultatory or echocardiographic evidence of MVP. They base their recommendations on the angiographic picture and on the report of endocarditis in one patient with papillary muscle dysfunction and mitral regurgitation. I strongly disagree with this recommendation because, to my knowledge, association between endocarditis and angiographic MVP, a nonspecific finding in coronary artery disease, has not been described.

SUDDEN DEATH IN MVP

Sudden death, the most feared complication of idiopathic MVP, is fortunately a rare occurrence. To my knowledge, only 25 cases of sudden death, including four of mine, have been reported (8,18,26,73,149,150,154, 175,201,239,253,290,332,364,384) (Table 14.2). Another group of 21 patients sustained ventricular fibrillation and were successfully resuscitated (51,53,73,175,228,253,301,341,380,386). Judging from cases of sudden death, mentioned by medical audiences during discussion of MVP, it would seem that a larger number of patients with sudden death goes unreported. Moreover, in familial studies in MVP (17,18,334) unexplained sudden death has been reported in relatives of the propositi. In long term follow-up studies covering 373 patients with a mean follow-up time of 4 to 20 years, only nine cases of sudden death and one case of successfully resuscitated ventricular fibrillation were reported (Table 14.1). One-half of these cases have been reported by one group (201). All of these series have originated from cardiology centers where patients with symptoms and EKG abnormalities are referred and are not, therefore, representative of this prevalent syndrome as seen in the general population. In my series of 32 patients reported in 1971 (169), four sudden deaths occurred; two had died before 1971 and were included retrospectively and the remaining two have died since publication.

The following is a brief case report of the four patients I have observed (175,278,384).

CASE REPORTS

Case 1

A 62-year-old woman with the chief complaint of moderate dyspnea with episodes of paroxysmal nocturnal dyspnea for which she was digitalized was followed in our cardiac clinic; there was no history of chest pain. An isolated pansystolic murmur was heard. The electrocardiogram showed atrial fibrillation, multiple PVC's, T wave inversion in I,II, AVF and V_4–V_6 and evidence of left ventricular hypertrophy; the Q-T interval was 34 msec. Chest films showed moderate cardiomegaly. Cardiac catheterization revealed the following data: pulmonary artery pressure, 26/16; "PC", 13 mmHg mean; left ventricular pressure, 125/12 and a cardiac index of 2.2 liters/m/M$_2$. On left ventriculography (Fig. 12.17) there was prolapse of both leaflets with a doughnut-like appearance, increased left ventricular contractility, and moderate mitral regurgitation. The patient died in her sleep. At necropsy both mitral leaflets were voluminous and redundant, the chordae were intact, and extensive myxomatous transformation of the mitral cusps was observed. There was evidence of minimal coronary artery disease. The patient's daughter had a midsystolic click and late systolic murmur and her grandson had multiple clicks.

Case 2

A 44-year-old woman died suddenly 3 years after cardiac catheterization. A murmur was heard for the first time at age 12. Her chief complaints were exertional chest pain, moderate dyspnea, lightheadedness, and attacks of near syncope. She was on digitalis. A Grade IV/VI apical pansystolic murmur with late systolic accentuation was heard. Electrocardiogram showed atrial fibrillation, multiple

PVC's, and T wave inversion in the inferior and left precordial leads. The Q-T interval was 32 msec. Chest X-ray films showed slight cardiomegaly and slight left atrial enlargement. Cardiac catheterization findings were as follows: pulmonary artery pressure, 27/12 with a mean of 18 mmHg; "PC", 14 mmHg mean, with a V wave of 21 mmHg; left ventricular pressure, 115/12; cardiac index 3.63 liters/m/M_2. Left ventriculography revealed massive prolapse of both leaflets and a voluminous doughnut-like appearance with a prominent anterior hump (Fig. 12.19). A cleft of radionegativity between the two leaflets was noted, and moderate mitral insufficiency was present. Coronary arteriography was not performed. Necropsy studies were not carried out.

Case 3

A 40-year-old man died suddenly at his work desk on April 11, 1973. I had last seen him in 1964 for chest pain, palpitations, lightheadedness, attacks of presyncope, and atrial fibrillation; digitalis was administered. A pansystolic murmur with late systolic accentuation was heard, but no click was noted. The electrocardiogram revealed atrial fibrillation, multiple premature ventricular beats, normal Q-T interval, T wave inversion in Leads I, II, AVF, V_4–V_6, and left ventricular hypertrophy. Chest X-ray films showed mild to moderate cardiomegaly. Left ventriculography showed massive mitral valve prolapse (Fig. 14.9) and moderately severe to severe mitral regurgitation. On cardiac catheterization, the pulmonary artery pressure was 20/10 with a mean of 14, the "PC" pressure was 10mmHg mean, the left ventricular pressure 125/14 and the cardiac index, 2.4 liters/m/M_2. No autopsy was performed.

Case 4

A 39-year-old woman was found unconscious on June 27, 1974 by her husband, who initiated cardiopulmonary resuscitation. In the emergency room, she was found to have ventricular fibrillation and, although conversion to normal sinus rhythm was accomplished, she died 2 days later of irreversible brain damage. She had been essentially asymptomatic according to her husband and her only medication had been Lasix,® which was self administered for "fluid retention." The serum potassium level on admission was 3 mEq/liter. Multiple systolic clicks and a Grade III/VI late systolic murmur were heard and recorded in 1965. The electrocardiogram had revealed normal sinus rhythm, no premature ventricular beats, a normal Q-T interval and T wave inversion in Leads II, III and AVF. Chest X-ray films had shown a normal sized heart. Cardiac catheterization (1965) had revealed a pulmonary artery pressure of 20/6 with a mean of 10mmHg, a "PC" pressure of 7mmHg, a left ventricular pressure of 103/8 and a cardiac index of 2.5 liters/m/M_2. Left cineventriculography had shown mitral valve prolapse and mild mitral insufficiency. At autopsy both mitral leaflets were redundant, hooded, and myxomatous (Fig. 3.1). Her two children, aged 16 and 14 years, respectively, had acoustically "silent" mitral valve proven by echocardiography.

Summary of Findings in the 25 Reported Cases (Table 14.2)

Family history, provided in five reported cases, revealed sudden death in one family, and evidence of MVP in four other families. The sex of the patient was noted in 16 out of 25 reported cases and 11 of the 16 (69%)

TABLE 14.2. Sudden death in MVP data on 25 reported cases

Case Number and author	Sex	Age	Symptoms	Family history of MVP and/or sudden death	Electrocardiograms					Auscultation and Phonocardiograms
					Rhythm	QT interval	ST-T abnormalities	Arrhythmias		
Hancock (154)	F	30	Palpitations	NI	NSR	Prolonged ? Quinidine effect	T inversion V_1–V_5 and inferior leads	Frequent multifocal PVC's		MSC-LSM
Barlow (18)	M	39	NI	NI	NI	NI	NI	NI		MSC-LSM
Trent (364)	F	63	Palpitations Syncope Dyspnea Heart failure	NI	NSR	NI	ST-T Abnormalities in limb and lateral precordial leads	Occasional PVC's		LSM
Shappell (332)	F	27	Syncope	sudden death	NSR	Prolonged	T inversion in inferior leads	PVC's		MSC-LSM
Marshall (239)	F	36	Palpitations associated with slight faintness	MVP	NI	NI	NI	NI		NI
Jeresaty (175)	F	62	Dyspnea	MVP	AF	Normal	T inversion left precordial and inferior leads	PVC's		PM
Jeresaty (175)	F	44	Dyspnea Chest pain Near syncope	NI	AF	Normal	LVH-T inversion left precordial and inferior leads	Multiple PVC's		PM

TABLE 14.2. (Continued)

Case Number and author	Drugs at time of death	Chest x-ray films	Echocardiogram	Catheterization data	Angiographic data	Coronary Arteriography	Pathological data[a]	Miscellaneous
Hancock (154)	Quinidine	Normal	NP	NP	NP	NP	No cardiac abnormalities[a]	Died while mowing his lawn
Barlow (18)	NI	NI	NP	NP	NP	NP	Normal cor. art. voluminous posterior leaflet	Died 2 days after catheterization
Trent (364)	None	Slight LV enlargement	NP	Normal	Prolapse of middle scallop, MR	NP	NI on CA prolapse of posterior leaflet myxomatous degeneration	
Shappell (332)	Propranolol	Normal	NP	Normal	MVP	Normal	Prolapse of both leaflets myxomatous degeneration, normal CA	Died during an argument
Marshall (239)	None	NI	NP	NP	NP	NP	Prolapse of both leaflets, myxomatous degeneration normal cor. art.	Severe hemorrhoidal pain prior to death
Jeresaty (175)	Digitalis	2+/4+ Cardiomegaly	NP	LVEDP 12	Prolapse both leaflets mild MR	NP	Prolapse both leaflets, mild coronary artery disease	Died in her sleep
Jeresaty (175)	Digitalis	Mild cardiomegaly	NP	LVEDP 12	Massive prolapse both leaflets 2-3+ MR	NP	No necropsy	

TABLE 14.2. (Continued)

Case Number and author	Drugs at time of death	Chest x-ray films	Echocardiogram	Catheterization data	Angiographic data	Coronary Arteriography	Pathological data	Miscellaneous
Rakowski (156)	Died after self withdrawal of Propranolol and Phenobarbital	NI	NI	NI	MVP	NI		Death resulted from ventricular fibrillation
Belardi (26)	NI	NI	NI	NI	MVP no significant MR	Normal	NI	
Belardi (26)	NI	NI	NI	NI	MVP, no significant MR	Normal	NI	
Koch (201)	NI	NI	NI	NI	NI	NI	No coronary artery disease	
Koch (201)	NI	NI	NI	NI	NI	NI	No coronary artery disease	
Koch (201)	NI	NI	NI	NI	NI	NI	No coronary artery disease	
Koch (201)	NI	NI	NI	NI	NI	NI	No coronary artery disease	
Cobbs (73)	Propranolol	NI	NI	NI	NI	NI	Minimal fibrosis of papillary muscle marked myxomatous involvement of both leaflets	Died suddenly following a tennis game
Mills (253)	Quinidine started 48 hours before death	Progressive cardiomegaly	MVP	NP	NP	NP	Prolapse of both leaflets, MD, no CAD	Died suddenly at home

NI, no information; NP, not performed; MSC, midsystolic click; LSM, late systolic murmur; NSR, normal sinus rhythm; PVC, premature ventricular contractions; PAC, premature atrial contractions; AF, atrial fibrillation; CA, coronary arteries; N, normal; MR, mitral regurgitation; MD, myxomatous degeneration; LVEDP, left ventricular end diastolic pressure; CAD, coronary artery disease.

[a] At autopsy performed elsewhere no cardiac or other abnormalities were reported.
[b] Cardiac catheterization nine years earlier.
[c] Cardiac catheterization nine years earlier.
[d] Diffuse interstitial fibrosis of inferobasilar wall of the left ventricle.
[e] Minimal interstitial fibrosis in the posterobasilar subendocardial area.

TABLE 14.2. (*Continued*)

Case Number and author	Sex	Age	Symptoms	Family history of MVP and/or sudden death	Electrocardiograms			Arrhythmias	Auscultation and Phonocardiograms
					Rhythm	QT interval	ST-T abnormalities		
Rakowski (156)	NI	NI	? Syncope	NI	NI	NI	NI	Required de-fibrillator	NI
Belardi (26)	NI	NI	NI	NI	NI	NI	NI	NI	NI
Belardi (26)	NI	NI	NI	NI	NI	NI	NI	NI	NI
Koch (201)	NI	9	NI	NI	NI	NI	NI	Two of Koch's four patients had multifocal PVC's	
Koch (201)	NI	32	NI	NI	NI	NI	NI		
Koch (201)	NI	50	NI	NI	NI	NI	NI		
Koch (201)	NI	64	NI	NI	NI	NI	NI		
Cobbs (73)	M	31	NI	NI	NI	NI	NI	Multiple PVC's	MSC-LSM
Mills (253)	M	58	Left ventricular failure	NI	AF	NI	ST-T changes	PVC's after cardioversion	LSM

TABLE 14.2. (Continued)

Case Number and author	Sex	Age	Symptoms	Family history of MVP and/or sudden death	Rhythm	QT interval	ST-T abnormalities	Arrhythmias	Auscultation and Phonocardiograms
							Electrocardiograms		
Jeresaty (384)	M	40	Near syncope, chest pain, palpitations, heart failure	NI	AF	Normal	LVH, T wave inversion left precordial and inferior leads	Multiple PVC's	PM
Jeresaty (384)	F	39	Asymptomatic ? water retention	"silent" MVP by echo in both children	NSR	Normal	T wave inversion inferior leads	No PVC's	MSC-LSM 9 years earlier
Guthrie and Edwards (384)	M	29	Asymptomatic	NI	NSR	NI	NI	PVC's, one episode of supraventricular tachycardia	PM
Guthrie and Edwards (384)	F	25	Syncope, chest pain fatigue, dyspnea, palpitations	NI	NSR	NI	NI	Multiple PVC's	MSC-LSM
Guthrie and Edwards (384)	F	20	Asymptomatic	NI	NSR	Normal	none	Frequent PVC's and PAC's	"Faint click at the base" no murmur
Gulotta (149)	F	53	Chest pain	NI	NSR	Normal	T wave inversion V_3–V_6 during pain only	PAC, PVC on exertion	MSC-LSM
Appblatt (8)	F	46	NI	NI	NI	NI	NI	NI	NI
Sorensen (341)	NI	54	NI	NI	NI	NI	NI	NI	NI
Rakowski (156)	NI	NI	Syncope	NI	NI	NI	NI	"Required a defibrillator"	NI

TABLE 14.2. (Continued)

Case Number and author	Drugs at time of death	Chest x-ray films	Echocardiogram	Catheterization data	Angiographic data	Coronary Arteriography	Pathological data	Miscellaneous
Jeresaty (384)	Digitalis	Mild to moderate cardiomegaly	NP	LVEDP 14	Massive prolapse both leaflets 2+ MR[b]	NP	No necropsy	Died at his work desk
Jeresaty (384)	Lasix	Normal	NP	LVEDP 8[c]	Mild MR prolapsed posterior leaflet	NP	Massive prolapse both leaflets, MD, normal coronary arteries	Found unconscious by husband K = 3 meq/liter
Guthrie and Edwards (384)	NI	NI	NP	NP	NP	NP	MVP both leaflets, MD, mild coronary atherosclerosis, friction lesions[d]	Died while working at desk
Guthrie and Edwards (384)	? Quinidine, high dose of Propanolol	NI	NP	NP	MVP, mild MR	NP	MVP both leaflet, MD, friction lesions[e]	Epicardial pacemaker Died 1 day after discharge fm hospital
Guthrie and Edwards (384)	None	NI	NP	NP	NP	NP	Normal sized heart MVP	PVC's disappear on exertion
Gulotta (149)	NI	NI	NP	LVEDP 8 C.I.-2.2	2+ MVP 1+ MR	Normal	NA	NI
Appblatt (8)	NI	NI	NI	NI	NI	NI	NI	NI
Sorensen (341)	NI	NI	NI	NI	NI	NI	NI	No significant coronary artery disease
Rakowski (156)	None	NI	NI	NI	MVP	NI	NI	Death resulted from ventricular fibrillation

were females. The age, reported in 21 patients, ranged from 9 to 23 years with a mean of 40.5 years. Death occurred during physical or emotional stress in four patients and at rest in seven. Information on symptoms was available in 15 patients, of whom five had chest pain, six had dyspnea and five had palpitations; syncope or near syncope was more prevalent, having occurred in eight patients. Auscultatory and phonocardiographic findings were reported in 14 patients; only one of these 14 had an isolated click described as "a very faint systolic click at the base" (Case 12 in Table 14.2). A late systolic murmur heard in nine patients, was preceded by a nonejection click in seven, and a pansystolic murmur was heard in four.

Adequate electrocardiographic information was provided for 12 patients with mention of arrhythmias in six other patients. Of the 12 patients, eight were in normal sinus rhythm and four in atrial fibrillation. PVC's, reported in 14 out of 18 patients in whom information on arrhythmias was available, were often described as frequent and multifocal. Three patients had had successful defibrillation of previous episodes of ventricular fibrillation (201, 332). Bradyarrhythmias were not described. The Q-T interval, mentioned in eight patients, was prolonged in only two. The Q-T interval prolongation in one of these two patients was probably quinidine-induced (Case 1 in Table 14.2). ST-T wave abnormalities were noted in nine patients. Since only two patients were on quinidine at the time of death and one was probably on quinidine, "quinidine syncope" cannot be invoked as a major cause of death in these patients. In only one patient (Case 25) in whom it was started 48 hr prior to demise could quinidine be probably incriminated. Three patients were on digitalis and three on propranolol. In one patient (Case 11) an epicardial pacemaker had been implanted to allow the use of high doses of propranolol which had resulted in marked bradycardia. Hemodynamic data were available in only seven patients and did not reveal significant disturbances: left ventricular end-diastolic pressure was elevated in only one patient. Coronary arteriography performed in four patients showed no abnormalities. Of nine patients whose coronary arteries were examined at necropsy only two had coronary artery disease and in both it was mild (one of these 9 patients had coronary arteriography and the normal arteriographic findings were confirmed at necropsy). Therefore, only two of 12 patients had coronary artery disease and the disease was mild in both. Left ventriculography, performed in 12 patients, demonstrated MVP in all; mild to moderate mitral regurgitation was demonstrated in nine.

Necropsy examination of the mitral valve was carried out in 12 patients (Figs. 3.1, 3.3, 3.4, and 12.9) and showed redundant, hooded, and myxomatous leaflets in all but in one case in which the autopsy was "performed elsewhere" (Case 1). Both leaflets were involved in the great majority of these cases. No myocardial abnormalities were noted except for friction lesions in two patients and interstitial fibrosis in the papillary muscles and the inferobasilar subendocardial areas in three (Cases 3, 10, and 11).

From a review of these 25 cases of fatal MVP, a composite picture of the possible candidate for sudden death emerges (156): a forty-year-old woman, with a history of syncopal or presyncopal episodes, who has a late systolic murmur preceded by a click, or a pansystolic murmur with late systolic accentuation. The electrocardiogram shows ST–T changes in the left precordial and inferior leads and multiple PVC's. Left ventriculography displays pronounced MVP with involvement of both leaflets and minimal to moderate mitral regurgitation (Fig. 12.17, 12.19, and 14.9). It is of interest that in patients who experienced ventricular fibrillation and were successfully resuscitated there was a high prevalence of late systolic murmur. Late systolic murmur with or without a click was noted in eight out of ten patients in whom auscultatory information was provided versus only two with isolated clicks. Repolarization abnormalities were also quite common (five out of five) and PVC's were prevalent (seven out of seven).

Sudden death has not been reported in "silent" MVP and it has been reported in only one patient with isolated click. Therefore, patients with MVP and late or pansystolic murmur are at a higher risk of dying suddenly (253) as they are of developing other complications including ruptured chordae tendineae and bacterial endocarditis. Patients with "silent" MVP or isolated click do not seem to incur these dramatic complications.

In view of the reports of sudden death in young relatives of propositi in familial studies of MVP, and of the relatively high occurrence of MVP in families of patients who died suddenly, it is possible that the familial forms of MVP carry a higher risk of sudden death.

Mechanism of Sudden Death

The mechanism of sudden death is probably arrhythmic. In MVP, which is frequently associated with PVC's, PAC's, and occasionally with ventricular tachycardia, ventricular fibrillation has been documented both in patients who have died suddenly and in those who were successfully resuscitated. Bradyarrhythmias that have been postulated as a possible mechanism of sudden death in this syndrome (217) have not been documented in any of the reported patients who have died suddenly. The relatively frequent occurrence of preexcitation in MVP and the demonstration of concealed bypass tracts in this syndrome (183) offer a possible explanation for the ventricular fibrillation in this syndrome, e.g., rapid transmission of atrial flutter or fibrillation across the bypass tracts leading to ventricular fibrillation (atrioventricular fibrillation). This mechanism was documented in one patient with MVP during a syncopal episode (51). Preexcitation has not been described in patients who have died suddenly.

Since cerebral embolism originating from fibrin deposits on the redundant leaflets has been postulated to explain TIA associated with MVP (21), it is remotely possible that coronary arterial embolism occurs in this syndrome and may be a rare mechanism of sudden death.

A review of coronary arteriographic and pathological findings (Table

14.2) would indicate a striking absence of coronary artery disease. This disease cannot, therefore, be incriminated as a cause of sudden death in these patients. Furthermore, there is no evidence to indicate that the angiographic MVP frequently noted in patients with coronary artery disease increases the risk of sudden death in these patients. This is an expected finding since MVP in coronary artery disease is pathogenically different from the idiopathic myxomatous prolapse.

Hypokalemia may be a contributory factor in the development of ventricular tachycardia and fibrillation in this syndrome. It was noted in one of our patients (Case 4) and in others who have developed life-threatening arrhythmias (386). Winkle et al. (386) reported electrolyte abnormalities or change in medications known to affect myocardial repolarization during the week before the episode in three of four patients with cardiac arrest. They felt that potassium wasting diuretics should be used prudently, and that the possible role of hypokalemia in life-threatening ventricular arrhythmia in MVP should be kept in mind. As initial treatment for ventricular irritability, they favored propranolol rather than quinidine and procainamide because "the latter drugs were more likely to increase the frequently existing myocardial repolarization abnormality." As mentioned above, quinidine was used in only three patients who died suddenly.

Treatment of Arrhythmias in MVP for Prevention of Sudden Death

MVP is recognized as a prevalent syndrome, but only 25 cases of sudden death and 14 cases of successful ventricular defibrillation have been reported in this syndrome. Although sudden death is primarily a risk in patients who show frequent PVC's, it should be considered as a rare occurrence, even in this subgroup, since PVC's are common in MVP. The rare occurrence of sudden death would not warrant aggressive antiarrhythmic therapy in all patients with MVP who exhibit ventricular irritability. The management of arrhythmias in this syndrome was reviewed in Chap. 8.

From the published data, I have identified a subgroup of patients at a higher risk of sudden death: patients with recurrent episodes of syncope, repolarization abnormalities, multiple PVC's, and late or pansystolic murmur. In these patients aggressive antiarrhythmic management is probably warranted. Patients with mitral regurgitation as evidenced by a late or pansystolic murmur represent a subgroup prone to complications and deserve particular attention (253) when they present with a history of syncope and palpitations and their rest EKG or Holter monitor display multiple PVC's and repolarization abnormalities.

The risk of sudden death, although remote, may have to be taken into account in weighing surgical indications in patients with MVP and severe mitral regurgitation; it may tilt the balance in favor of surgery in this difficult decision.

In evaluating the cause of sudden death, particularly in young women, both general and forensic pathologists "should maintain a high index of suspicion that the death may be related to the ballooning posterior leaflet syndrome" (239). By overlooking the myxomatous mitral changes, grossly and microscopically, there is "a chance that the autopsy may be interpreted as revealing no anatomic cause of death" (150).

In conclusion, the risk of sudden death is remote in this syndrome and, therefore, should not be mentioned to the patient or his family for fear of inducing undue anxiety and neurosis (384). The occurrence of this dramatic complication. albeit rare, indicates that this syndrome is not always benign.

Chapter 15

Surgical Treatment of MVP

Cardiac surgery is mainly performed in the advanced form of idiopathic MVP, the "floppy" valve syndrome (77,244,319). It is also carried out when ruptured chordae tendineae had supervened and had resulted in rapid or gradual deterioration. The damage wreaked upon the prolapsed valve by endocarditis often requires surgical intervention. In a few cases, cardiac surgery was carried out for intractable ventricular arrhythmias with recurrent ventricular fibrillation and for intractable chest pain.

Mitral valve replacement is the most widely used cardiac surgical intervention in MVP. At this time, plication, annuloplasty, or reattachment of ruptured chordae tendineae are rarely performed. Recently one group (78, 395) used a posterior annular collar prosthesis for surgical repair in symptomatic MVP.

MITRAL VALVE REPLACEMENT FOR SEVERE MITRAL REGURGITATION IN MVP

The myxomatous "floppy" mitral valve is now recognized as a major cause of mitral insufficiency (77,229,244,297,319). Associated chordal rupture is frequently noted on surgical exploration. It is estimated that mitral valve replacement for "floppy" mitral valve accounts for one-tenth of all valve replacements (108,244) and that the "floppy" mitral valve accounts for one-fourth (77) to one-half (319) of mitral valve replacement for pure mitral insufficiency.

The first reported large series (77) of surgery on mitral regurgitation due to "floppy valve syndrome" consisted of 50 patients. Nineteen of these patients had ruptured chordae tendineae. Various valve prostheses were used. The operative mortality was 10% (5 of 50) and four of these five patients died "as a result of recurrent dehiscence of the mitral prosthesis." There were eight late deaths, one as a result of dehiscence. Most of these prostheses were fixed by a continuous suture technique. In a second large series of 38 patients, employing fresh aortic homografts (244) the 30-day operative mortality was 10.5%. There were two late deaths, both sudden over a follow-up period of as long as 36 months. Ruptured chordae tendineae was noted in 31 patients. These authors recommended mitral valve replacement "soon after the onset of congestive heart failure." Valve dehiscence did not occur in this series. In a third series of 66 patients (319), the operative mortality (less than 30 days) was 6% (38 Starr Edwards prosthesis and 28 xenografts or allografts). The late postoperative survival rate ($53 \pm 8\%$ 5-year survival) in this series was unusually low in comparison with the group's general experience for isolated mitral valve replacement and "illustrates the relatively serious nature of this disorder" (319). A highly significant impact of advanced functional disability (New York Heart Association Class IV) on survival was demonstrated. Ruptured chordae tendineae was noted in 41 patients. Seven of 21 late postoperative deaths were due to congestive heart failure, five were sudden and unexplained, and three were caused by documented ventricular arrhythmias. Partial valve dehiscence occurred in two patients, and in both reoperation was necessary to close perivalvular leak.

These three series document the frequency of "floppy" mitral valve as a cause of mitral regurgitation and the prevalence of ruptured chordae tendineae in this entity. Dehiscence of the valve prothesis is a complication of mitral valve replacement, particularly when a rigid prosthesis is used (77, 297,313). It was not observed in the one series that used fresh aortic homograft (244) and in another series of 12 cases (229) in which mechanical prostheses were used. In another series of 66 patients, dehiscence was noted in only two (319). A high dehiscence rate was reported by one group (77) who used continuous sutures in most of their patients but recommended interrupted rather than continuous suture to avoid impairing the blood supply to the annulus. The annulus, when involved by the myxomatous process does not hold sutures as well as the fibrotic annulus of rheumatic valvular disease and accounts for the relative high incidence of dehiscence in patients with "floppy" mitral valve.

The preoperative diagnosis of "floppy" mitral valve and its recognition at surgery are important to the surgeon because these patients display a tendency to disruption of suture lines with displacement of prosthesis (297). Surgeons should exercise special care during valve replacement to lessen the likelihood of dehiscence. Several operative techniques have been described to prevent this problem (157) and include the use of interrupted rather than continuous sutures (77), the use of Teflon pledgets to support sutures, the placement of the prosthesis below the mitral annulus (130), vertical mattress sutures (157), and finally more sutures than normal in mitral valve replacement.

The impact of myxomatous MVP on late postoperative mortality requires further study. In most series, the late mortality seems to be high in comparison with the general experience for isolated mitral valve replacement (319). Many of these deaths were sudden raising the question of their relationship to the arrhythmias commonly observed in this syndrome. However, as pointed out by Salomon et al. (319), late postoperative sudden death is not unique to patients undergoing mitral valve replacement for myxomatous disease. There is a definite need to compare prospectively the prevalence of

immediate and late postoperative arrhythmias and sudden death in patients
with "floppy" mitral valve and mitral regurgitation to that in patients undergoing mitral valve replacement for other types of heart disease particularly
rheumatic heart disease. This type of study would determine whether an
aggressive long-term antiarrhythmic regimen should be recommended in
MVP patients. If such studies should document a higher incidence of arrhythmias and sudden death then an explanation for these findings should
be sought. Proponents of the myocardial theory of MVP would not be surprised by this finding whereas proponents of the valvular theory would have
to postulate persistence of secondary endomyocardial fibrosis to account for
the persistence of arrhythmias.

Some workers (130,244,296,297) reported frequent occurrence of associated aortic valve disease in "floppy" mitral syndrome. Dilatation of the aortic
ring and mucinous degeneration of the aortic cusps themselves have been
described (244). The cusps were soft and thin with slightly thickened edges
and tended to prolapse. The resulting severe aortic insufficiency required
aortic valve replacement. Frable (130) reported severe isolated aortic insufficiency requiring surgery in seven patients with prosthetic valve dehiscence
occurring in three. Others (77,319), in two series with a total of 116 patients
with "floppy" mitral valve, have reported myxomatous transformation of the
aortic valve requiring aortic valve replacement in only one patient (77). I
noted aortic insufficiency of minimal severity in only two of my patients.
None of our eleven patients who underwent mitral valve replacement for
"floppy" mitral valve had associated aortic insufficiency.

In addition to prosthetic dehiscence, acute aortic dissection during mitral
valve replacement for "floppy" mitral valve has been reported (244,245).
Dissection was due to application of aortic clamp to the ascending aorta
during cardiopulmonary bypass. The ascending aorta appeared grossly normal
and "histological examination revealed areas of elastic disruption or mucoid
degeneration" (245). The authors suggested infrequent clamping of the
aorta and control of the perfusion pressure to decrease the risk of intimal
trauma and acute dissection.

SURGICAL TREATMENT OF "FLOPPY" MITRAL
VALVE IN CHILDREN

Sherman et al. (335) were the first to report mitral valve replacement for
"floppy" mitral valve and severe mitral regurgitation in children. Their patient, an eight-year-old black girl was still doing well one year postoperatively.
A Japanese group (115) performed mitral valve replacement in five children
ranging in age from nine to 14 years. The clinical course in this age group
was characterized by rapid deterioration in heart failure after the onset of
symptoms. Three out of the five patients required tricuspid valve replacement
for a "floppy" tricuspid valve. The authors recommended early surgical

treatment after the onset of heart failure in children with "floppy" mitral valve. They have postulated a racial difference in the progress of this syndrome. Mitral insufficiency in Marfan's syndrome in children tend to progress rapidly (115).

CARDIAC SURGERY FOR RELIEF OF PAIN AND INTRACTABLE ARRHYTHMIAS IN MVP

Mitral valve replacement has been used for relief of intractable chest pain in one patient (224). Recently Cooley et al. (78,395) have used a posterior annular collar prosthesis for relief of symptoms. In this operation, the prolapsed scallop of the posterior leaflet is retracted, the redundant central portion is excised, and the created defect is repaired with interrupted sutures, obliterating the redundancy of the posterior leaflet. A C ring prosthesis made of Dacron ribbon and covered with Dacron velour fabric is inserted beginning at the anterior lateral commissure. The insertion is completed with individual mattress sutures reinforced with Teflon pledglets. In this operation, the need for mitral valve replacement is obviated (See Chapter 5).

Mitral valve replacement has been performed in five patients for prevention of recurrent ventricular tachycardia and fibrillation resistant to antiarrhythmic therapy (73,175,380) (See Chapter 8).

In summary, myxomatous transformation of the mitral valve is a major cause of pure mitral insufficiency. Severe mitral regurgitation is the only accepted indication for cardiac surgery and mitral valve replacement. There is a relatively high incidence of valve dehiscence presumably due to myxomatous changes in the annulus. This risk can be minimized by careful surgical techniques. Longterm survival rates in these patients is lower in comparison to other groups undergoing mitral valve replacement. The mechanism for this high late mortality has not been elucidated.

Chapter 16

Conclusion, Personal Views, and Future Directions

Idiopathic MVP has emerged, during the past decade, as the most common valvular disorder probably affecting about 4% of the population. In this book I have strived to present, as objectively as possible, the various theories which have been proposed to explain the etiology and the various features of this intriguing syndrome. When presented with conflicting information, the author of a book on a recently described entity is expected to "editorialize" and to state his own views. In the preceding chapters, I have already expressed my "bias" in discussing various aspects of this syndrome. I hope, at this point, to summarize my views and to stress areas that are ripe for future investigations.

The etiology of this syndrome has not been fully unraveled, but the overwhelming evidence points to myxomatous transformation of the mitral valve as the underlying pathological abnormality. Characteristically, the mitral cusps are voluminous and redundant. Myocardial involvement is probably a secondary phenomenon. Further study will probably confirm a coincidental rather than a causal relationship between coronary artery disease and idiopathic MVP, two common entities. The nature of the myxomatous process, its basic histology, histo-chemistry, and particularly its relationship to connective tissue disorders deserve in depth investigation. These studies will probably detect a gradation from a normal mitral valve, to a minimally deformed valve, as a normal variant, to a moderately involved valve associated with a click and/or late systolic murmur and finally to a severely damaged valve e.g. the "floppy" valve (Table 3.1). The "silent" form may be the earliest phase of a "continuum" and the "floppy" valve the end of the spectrum. Further follow-up studies are required to document a transition from one form to the other and the possible mechanism responsible for "freezing" in one group as opposed to rapid progression and deterioration in another. The "floppy" valve is now recognized as the major cause of mitral regurgitation but many gaps are still evident in its natural history. Is the "floppy" mitral valve, which is observed in the middle aged and the elderly patients, preceded by "silent" prolapse, a nonejection click or a late systolic murmur at a younger age? This transition has not been definitely documented. It is of interest, however, that the most benign and the most severe form of idiopathic MVP share the same myxomatous process, albeit of a variable severity, and the same echocardiographic and angiographic features.

This syndrome is probably a more common cause of chest pain than other etiologies which are invoked to explain chest pain in the absence of coronary artery disease. The chest pain can be disabling and intractable and its relief remains a challenge for further investigation. The psychiatric manifestations of this syndrome, their true prevalence and significance await further studies. Are they actually more prevalent in this syndrome than in the general population and are they a manifestation of a systemic disorder which includes thoracic skeletal abnormalities, pulmonary emphysema, dermatoglyphic anomalies, secundum atrial septal defect, and so forth?

The auscultatory manifestations of this syndrome have been the subject of excellent clinical studies. The "silent" form, its prevalence and its significance should be further explored. Is it an echocardiographic or angiographic curiosity or could it be the harbinger of more serious complications? Long-term follow-up studies would provide the answer to these questions. I have repeatedly stressed the importance of nonejection click as the auscultatory "hallmark" of this syndrome. The click's underlying pathology (e.g., myxomatous transformation of the mitral valve) has been documented in only 26 cases. Pathological or surgical data on patients with nonejection clicks should be diligently sought and published to confirm these findings and to justify the belief held by many workers, including this author, that nonejection clicks, with a few exceptions, are due to myxomatous, redundant mitral cusps. The nonspecificity of the isolated late systolic murmur and the need for echocardiographic or angiographic confirmation of MVP when this finding is noted have been stressed in preceding chapters.

Repolarization abnormalities, atrial and ventricular arrhythmias are common in this syndrome and the rare occurrence of sudden death has been reported. It is my view that only symptomatic and life threatening arrhythmias should be treated. Further studies on the indications for antiarrhythmic therapy and the efficacy of various antiarrhythmic agents are urgently needed. False-positive stress tests are common in this syndrome and should be supplemented by thallium 201 scintigraphy to improve their specificity.

Echocardiography provides an invaluable noninvasive tool for the recognition of MVP. One of its features, midsystolic buckling, is almost specific of MVP but other features, particularly pansystolic sagging, suffer from nonspecificity and their significance is not clear at this time. Unfortunately, many echocardiographers are "overdiagnosing" a cardiac disease on the basis of unproven criteria. It is hoped that two-dimensional echocardiography may provide more meaningful diagnostic information.

The angiographic diagnosis of this syndrome suffers from nonspecificity of many of its features, from common occurrence of "normal variants" and from lack of quantitative data. Quantitation of angiographic prolapse and better definition of the "pathological" as opposed to "normal variants" are fertile grounds for further investigation. I have already stressed the frequent occurrence of nonspecific angiographic prolapse in coronary artery disease. This represents an incidental finding unrelated to mitral valve pathology and exhibiting a discordance with auscultatory and echocardiographic signs of MVP.

Of the associated disease, secundum atrial septal defect is one of the most common. It is possible that MVP has been overdiagnosed in ASD on the basis of the angiographic appearance which can mimic that which is associated with mitral valve pathology. Auscultatory and echocardiographic confirmation of MVP are required before the diagnosis of association of this entity with ASD is made.

The prognosis in this syndrome is probably benign. However, the occurrence of complications, albeit rare, including progression of mitral regurgitation, chordal rupture, infective endocarditis and sudden death have shattered the illusion of innocence of this syndrome. Patients with "silent" MVP or with isolated click are at a lower risk of major complications unlike those who suffer from mitral regurgitation manifested as a late or pansystolic murmur. Progression of mitral regurgitation and ruptured chordae tendineae are more common in males, clouding, therefore, the outlook in these patients.

Idiopathic MVP is being recognized as a major cause of isolated ruptured chordae tendineae. I believe that future clinical and pathological studies would prove MVP as the most common etiology of ruptured chordae tendinea even if chordal rupture due to superimposed endocarditis is excluded.

Infective endocarditis is an uncommon complication of MVP. In view of the rare occurrence of this complication and the side effects of antibiotics, the wisdom of antibiotic prophylaxis has been justifiably questioned. I do not believe that antibiotic prophylaxis is warranted in "silent" MVP or in isolated click, however, I would recommend antibiotics when a late or pansystolic murmur of mitral regurgitation are present. Further research based on randomized patients should be carried out to better define the indications for antibiotic prophylaxis in MVP.

The place of cardiac surgery in the management of intractable chest pain and intractable life threatening arrhythmias needs more study. I do not foresee a major role for cardiac surgery in this syndrome except as a treatment for severe mitral regurgitation. The problem of prosthesis dehiscence should benefit from advances in surgical technique.

Considerable investigation is needed to elucidate the various aspects of this interesting and yet poorly understood syndrome (175). I wish to conclude by quoting from a recent article by Dr. Michael Halberstam in the New York Times (152): "This is not to indicate despair at the state of modern medicine, only to recall how much mystery remains. Because of this, physicians will continue—must continue—to apply partially understood therapies to barely understood illness. It is foolish for critics of medicine to puff up righteously about "unproven therapies." Very little in medicine is proven. Diagnosis and treatment move haltingly, ahead a few steps here, back a few there, into blind alleys often enough. Breakthroughs are rare, increments common. The practicing physician learns to live with this frustration though not to enjoy it."

References

1. Abinader, E. G. (1976). Adrenergic beta blockade and ECG changes in the systolic click murmur syndrome. *Am. Heart J.,* 91:297–302.
2. Abinader, E. G. (1976): Mitral valve prolapse—Letter to the editor *Circulation,* 54:845–846.
3. Abrams, J. (1976): Mitral valve prolapse: A plea for unanimity. *Am. Heart J.* 92:413–415.
4. Ainsworth, R. P., Hartmann, A. F., Aker, U., et al. (1973): Tricuspid valve prolapse with late systolic tricuspid insufficiency. *Radiology,* 107:309–311.
5. Allen, H., Harris, A., Leatham, A. (1974): Significance and prognosis of an isolated late systolic murmur: A 9- to 22-year follow-up. *Br. Heart J.,* 36:525–532.
6. Antani, J., Srinivas, H. V. (1974): Cardiovascular abnormalities in Ehlers-Danlos syndrome. *Chest (abstr),* 65:5.
7. Antonelli, G., Brindicci, G., DiBiase, M., et al. (1976): Prolasso della mitrale e sindrome di pre-eccitazione ventricolare. *G. Ital. Cardiol.,* 6:1365–1377.
8. Appelblatt, N. H., Willis, P. W., Lenhart, J. A., et al. (1975): Ten to 40 year follow-up of 69 patients with systolic click with or without apical late systolic murmur. *Am. J. Cardiol. (abstr),* 35:119.
9. Applefeld, M. M., Bon Tempo, C. P., Ronan, J. A., et al. (1974): The effect of amyl nitrite on the murmur of mitral regurgitation. *Circulation (abstr),* 50 (suppl III):214.
10. Aranda, J. M.: (1976): Mitral valve prolapse—Letter to the editor. *Circulation,* 54:846.
11. Aranda, J. M., Befeler, B., El-Sherif, N., et al. (1976): Mitral valve prolapse. *Am. J. Med.,* 60:997–1004.
12. Aranda, J. M., Befeler, B., Lazzara, R., et al. (1975): Mitral valve prolapse and coronary artery disease. Clinical, hemodynamic, and angiographic correlations. *Circulation,* 52:245–253.
13. Aslam, P. A., Eastridge, C. E., Bernhardt, H., et al. (1970): Myxomatous degeneration of cardiac valves. *Chest,* 57:535–539.
14. Atlas, P., Yahini, J. H., Palant, A., et al. (1976): Chordal rupture: A common complication of myxomatous degeneration of the mitral valve. *Isr. J. Med. Sci.,* 12:1320–1324.
15. Awdeh, M., Gholston, D. E. (1977): Mitral valve prolapse and coronary artery spasm—Letter to the editor. *Circulation,* 56:329.
16. Barlow, J. B. (1976): Personal communication.
17. Barlow, J. B., Bosman, C. K. (1966): Aneurysmal protrusion of the posterior leaflet of the mitral valve. *Am. Heart J.,* 71:166–178.
18. Barlow, J. B., Bosman, C. K., Pocock, W. A., et al. (1968): Late systolic murmurs and non-ejection (mid-late) systolic clicks: An analysis of 90 patients. *Br. Heart J.,* 30:203–218.
19. Barlow, J. B., Pocock, W. A. (1975): The problem of nonejection systolic clicks and associated mitral systolic murmurs: Emphasis on the billowing mitral leaflet syndrome. *Am. Heart J.,* 90:636–655.
20. Barlow, J. B., Pocock, W. A., Marchand, P., et al. (1963): The significance of late systolic murmurs. *Am. Heart J.,* 66:443–452.
21. Barnett, H. J., Jones, M. W., Boughner, D. R., et al. (1976): Cerebral ischemic events associated with prolapsing mitral valve. *Arch. Neurol.,* 33:777–782.
22. Bashour, T., Lindsay, J. (1975): Midsystolic clicks originating from tricuspid valve structures: A sequela of heroin-induced endocarditis. *Chest,* 67:620–621.
23. Becker, A. E., Becker, M., Edwards, J. E. (1975): Mitral valvular abnormalities associated with supravalvular aortic stenosis. *Am. J. Cardiol.,* 29:90–94.

24. Becker, A. E., van Mantgem, J. P.: The coronary arteries in Marfan's syndrome. *Am. J. Cardiol.,* 36:315–321.

25. Behar, V. S., Whalen, R. E., McIntosh, H. D.: (1967): The ballooning mitral valve in patients with the "precordial honk" or "whoop." *Am. J. Cardiol.,* 20: 789–795.

26. Belardi, J., Lardani, H., Manubens, S., et al. (1976): Idiopathic prolapse of the mitral valve; a follow up study in 137 patients studied by angiography. *Am. J. Cardiol. (abstr),* 37:

27. Benchimol, A., Harris, C. L., Desser, K. B.: (1972): Midsystolic carotid pulse wave retraction in subjects with prolapsed mitral valve leaflets. *Chest,* 62:614–615.

28. Bensman, M., Delman, A., Cohen, M. V. (1975): Phonocardiographic follow-up of patients with late systolic murmur and/or midsystolic click. *Circulation (abstr),* 52 (Suppl II):159.

29. Betriu, A., Wigle, E. D., Felderhof, C. H., et al.: (1975): Prolapse of the posterior leaflet of the mitral valve associated with secundum atrial septal defect. *Am. J. Cardiol.,* 35:363–369.

30. Bharati, S., Lev, M. (1973): Congenital polyvalvular disease. *Circulation,* 48:575–585.

31. Bigger, J. T., Giardina, E. G. V., Perel, J. M., et al. (1977): Cardiac antiarrhythmic effect of imipramine hydrochloride. *New Engl. J. Med.,* 296:206–208.

32. Bittar, N., Sosa, J. A. (1968): The billowing mitral valve leaflet: Report on fourteen patients. *Circulation,* 38:763–770.

33. Bjerregaard, P., Peterson, E. L. C. (1977): Type A WPW and mitral valve prolapse—Letter to the editor. *Circulation,* 56:136–137.

34. Blieden, L. C., Desnick, R. J., Carter, J. B., et al.: (1974): Cardiac involvement in Sandhoff's disease. *Am. J. Cardiol.,* 34:83–88.

35. Blieden, L. C., Moller, J. (1974): Cardiac involvement in inherited disorders of metabolism. *Prog. Cardiovasc. Dis.,* 16:615–631.

36. Bloch, A., Vignola, P. A., Walker, H., Kaplan, A. D., Chiotellis, P. N., Lees, R. S., Myers, G. S. (1977): Echocardiographic spectrum of posterior systolic motion of the mitral valve in the general population. *J.C.U.,* 5:243–247.

37. Bonner, A. J., Noble, R. J., Feigenbaum, H., et al. (1976): Early diastolic sound associated with mitral valve prolapse. *Arch. Intern. Med.,* 136:347–349.

38. Bon Tempo, C. P., Ronan, J. A., deLeon, A. C., et al. (1975): Radiographic appearance of the thorax in systolic click-late systolic murmur syndrome. *Am. J. Cardiol.,* 36:27–31.

39. Boughner, D. R. (1975): Correlation of echocardiographic and angiographic abnormalities in mitral valve prolapse. *Ultrasound Med* I:55–62.

40. Brandt, K. D., Sumner, R. D., Ryan, T. J., et al. (1975): Herniation of mitral leaflets in the Ehlers-Danlos syndrome *Am. J. Cardiol.,* 36:524–528.

41. Brodsky, M., Wu, D., Denes, P., et al. (1977): Arrhythmias documented by 24 hour continuous electrocardiographic monitoring in 50 male medical students without apparent heart disease. *Am. J. Cardiol.,* 39:390–395.

42. Brown, D. D., Stoop, D. R., Stanton, K. C. (1973): Precipitation of cardiac arrhythmias in the mid-systolic click/late-systolic murmur syndrome by in-flight G_z maneuvers. *Aerospace Med.,* 44:1169–1172.

43. Brown, O. R., DeMots, H., Kloster, F. F., et al. (1975): Aortic root dilatation and mitral valve prolapse in Marfan's syndrome. *Circulation,* 52:651–657.

44. Brown, O. R., Kloster, F. E. (1975): Echocardiographic criteria for mitral valve prolapse. Effect of transducer position. *Circulation (abstr),* 51,52 (Suppl II):165.

45. Brown, O. R., Kloster, F. E., DeMots, H. (1975): Incidence of mitral valve prolapse in the asymptomatic normal. *Circulation (abstr),* 52 (Suppl 11):77.

46. Bulkley, B. H., Roberts, W. C. (1975): Dilatation of the mitral anulus. A rare cause of mitral regurgitation. *Am. J. Med.,* 59:457–463.

47. Burch, G. E., et al. (1968): The syndrome of papillary muscle dysfunction *Am. Heart J.,* 75:399.

48. Burggraf, G. W., Parker, J. C. (1974): Left ventricular volume changes after amyl nitrite and nitroglycerin in man as measured by ultrasound. *Circulation,* 49: 136–143.

49. Cabeen, W. R., Reza, M. J., Kovick, R. B., et al. (1977): Mitral valve prolapse and conduction defects in Ehlers-Danlos syndrome. *Arch. Intern. Med.,* 137:122–1231.

50. Call, T., Leier, C., Wooley, C. (1977): Cardiac defects in the Ehlers-Danlos syndrome. *Circulation,* 55,56 (Suppl III):69.

51. Camous, J. P., Guarino, L., Varenne, A., et al. (1977): Arythmie grave chez un sujet porteur d'une preexcitation ventriculaire et d'un prolapsus des deux valves mitrales. *Ann. Cardiol. Angeiol.,* 26:329–333.

52. Campbell, R. W. F., Godman, M. G., Fiddler, G. I., et al. (1976): Ventricular arrhythmias in the auscultatory-electrocardiographic variant of the balloon mitral valve syndrome. *Am. J. Cardiol. (abstr),* 37:126.

53. Campbell, R. W. F., Godman, M. G., Fiddler, G. I., et al. (1976): Ventricular arrhythmias in syndrome of balloon deformity of mitral valve definition of possible high risk group. *Br. Heart J.,* 38:1053–1057.

54. Case Records of the Massachusetts General Hospital (1967): *New Engl. J. Med.,* 277:92–101.

55. Case records of the Massachusetts General Hospital (1972): Floppy mitral valve and coronary artery fistula. *New Engl. J. Med.,* 287:456–462.

56. Case Records Massachusetts General Hospital (1974): *New Engl. J. Med.,* 290:330.

57. Case Records of the Massachusetts General Hospital (1974): *New Engl. J. Med.,* 290:617–623.

58. Case records of the Massachusetts General Hospital (1977): Mitral valve prolapse and idiopathic hypertrophic subaortic stenosis. *New Engl. J. Med.,* 297:1276–1283.

59. Caudill, C. C., Kruger, S. K., Wilson, C. S., et al. (1976): Membranous subaortic stenosis complicated by aneurysm of the membranous septum and mitral valve prolapse. *Circulation,* 53:580–583.

60. Cha, S. D., Gooch, A. S., Yang, S. S., et al. (1974): The vectorcardiogram in prolapsed mitral leaflet myocardiopathy. *J. Electrocardiol.,* 7:37–42.

61. Chandraratna, P. A. N. (1977): Limitations of the echocardiogram in diagnosing valvular vegetations in patients with mitral valve prolapse. *Circulation,* 56:436–438.

62. Chandraratna, P., Littman, B., Wilson, D. (1977): The association between atrial septal defect and tricuspid valve prolapse. *Chest (abstr),* 72:397.

63. Chandraratna, P. A., Lopez, J. M., Fernandex, J. J., et al. (1975): Echocardiographic detection of tricuspid valve prolapse. *Circulation,* 51:223–226.

64. Chandraratna, P. A. N., Lopez, J. M., Littman, B. B., et al. (1974): Abnormal mitral valve motion during ventricular extrasystoles: An echocardiographic study. *Am. J. Cardiol.,* 34:783–786.

65. Chandraratna, P. A. N., Tolentino, A. O., Mutucumarana, W., et al. (1977): Echocardiographic observations on the association between mitral valve prolapse and asymmetric septal hypertrophy. *Circulation,* 55:622–626.

66. Cheng, T. O. (1972): Late systolic murmur in coronary artery disease. *Chest,* 61:346–356.

67. Cheng, T. O. (1973): Midsystolic clicks and coronary heart disease—Letter to the editor. *Chest,* 63:298.

68. Cheng, T. O. (1976): The click-murmur syndrome—A medical pendulum and a unifying concept. *Chest,* 70:569–572.

69. Cheng, T. O. (1977): Diastolic click in mitral valve prolapse—Letter to the editor. *Arch. Intern. Med.,* 137:696.

70. Chesler, E., Matisonn, R. E., Lakier, J. B., et al. (1976): Acute myocardial infarction with normal coronary arteries. *Circulation,* 54:203–209.

71. Cobbs, B. W. Jr. (1974): In Hurst, J. W., Logue, R. B., Schlant, R. C., and Wenger, N. K. (eds.), *The Heart,* 3rd edition. McGraw-Hill, New York.

72. Cobbs, B. W., King, S. B. (1974): Mechanism of abnormal ventriculogram (VGM) and ECG associated with prolapsing mitral valve (MVP). *Circulation (abstr),* 49,50:

73. Cobbs, B. W., King, S. B. (1977): Ventricular buckling: A factor in the ab-

normal ventriculogram and peculiar hemodynamics associated with mitral valve prolapse. *Am. Heart J.,* 93:741–758.

74. Cohen, M. V. (1976): Double mitral leaflet prolapse: Echocardiographic phono-cardiographic correlation. *Am. Heart J.,* 91:168–177.

75. Cohn, I. H., Hultgren, H. N., Angell, W. W., et al. (1973): Prolapsing mitral valve with mucinous degeneration. *West. J. Med.,* 118:43–47.

76. Combs, R., Shah, P. M., Shulman, R., et al. (1977): Effects of psychological stress on click rhythm in mitral valve prolapse. *Circulation (abstr),* 55,56 (Suppl III):113.

77. Cooley, D. A., Gerami, S., Hallman, G. L., et al. (1972): Mitral insufficiency due to myxomatous transformation: "floppy valve syndrome. *J. Cardiovasc. Surg. (Torino),* 13:346–349.

78. Cooley, D. A., Frazier, O. H., Norman, J. C. (1976): Mitral leaflet prolapse: Surgical treatment using a posterior annular collar prosthesis *Cardiovasc. Dis. Bull. Texas Heart Institute,* 3:438–444.

79. Cowley, M. J., Coghlan, H. C., Mantle, J. A., et al. (1977): Chest pain and bi-lateral atrioventricular valve prolapse with normal coronary arteries in isolated corrected transposition of the great vessels. *Am. J. Cardiol.,* 40:458–462.

80. Corrigall, D., Bolen, J., Hancock, E., Popp, R. L. (1977): Mitral Valve Prolapse and infective endocarditis. *Am. J. Med.,* 63:215–222.

81. Cosby, R. S., Giddings, J. A., See J. R., et al. (1976): Late complications of myocardial infarction. *JAMA,* 236:1717–1720.

82. Craige, E. (1976): On the genesis of heart sounds. *Circulation,* 53:207–209.

83. Crawford, M. H. (1977): Mitral valve prolapse due to coronary artery disease. *Am. J. Med.,* 62:447–451.

84. Criley, J. M., Kissel, G. L. (1975): Prolapse of the mitral valve—the click and late systolic murmur syndrome. *Progr. Cardiology,* 4:23–36.

85. Criley, J. M., Lewis, K. B., Humphries, J. O., et al. (1966): Prolapse of the mitral valve: Clinical and cine-angiocardiographic findings. *Br. Heart J.,* 28:488–496.

86. Criley, J. M., Zeilenga, D. W., Morgan, M. T. (1973): Mitral dysfunction: A pos-sible cause of arrhythmias in the prolapsing mitral leaflet syndrome. *Trans. Am. Clin. Climatol. Assoc.,* 85:44–53.

87. Criscitiello, M. G., Ronan, J. A., Besterman, E. M. M., et al. (1965): Cardio-vascular abnormalities in osteogenesis imperfecta. *Circulation,* 31:255–262.

88. Cuffer, B. (1887): Nouvelles recherches sur le bruit galop. *Arch. Gen. Med.,* I:131–149, 301–320.

89. Daniels, D. H., D'Ambroso, U., Bedyned, J. (1974): Unusual abnormalities as-sociated with the floppy mitral valve syndrome. *Med. Ann. D. C.,* 43:4–8.

90. Dashkoff, N., Fortuin, N. J., Hutchins, G. M., et al. (1974): Clinical features of severe mitral regurgitation due to floppy valve. *Circulation (abstr),* 49,50 (Suppl III):60.

91. Davis, R. H., Schuster, B., Knoebel, S. B., et al. (1971): Myxomatous degenera-tion of the mitral valve. *Am. J. Cardiol.,* 28:449–455.

92. DeBusk, R. F., Harrison, D. C. (1969): The clinical spectrum of papillary muscle disease. *New Engl. Med.,* 281:1458–1467.

93. Deglin, J. M., Deglin, S. M. (1975): "Munchausen" case—Letter to the editor *Ann. Intern. Med.,* 82:721–722.

94. DeLezo, J. S., Garcia, E., Carrasco, J. L., et al. (1975): Quantitative segmental analysis of contractility in the prolapsed mitral valve syndrome measured by ejection indices. *Cardiovasc. Dis. Bull. Tex. Heart Inst.,* 2:

95. DelRio, C., Leatherman, I. L., Ambrust, C. A., et al., (1971): Chest pain and post-exercise ECG's with normal coronary arteriograms in patients with click-late systolic murmur syndrome. *Chest,* 60:292.

96. DeMaria, N., Bogren, H., Caudill, C. C., et al. (1975): Evaluation of the non-valvular factors of cardiac performance, left ventricular contractile pattern and coronary anatomy in the mitral valve prolapse syndrome. *Am. J. Cardiol. (abstr),* 35:132.

98. DeMaria, A. N., Amsterdam, E. A., Vismara, L. A., et al. (1976): the mitral valve prolapse syndrome. *Ann. Intern. Med.*, 84:656–660.

99. DeMaria, A. N., King, J. F., Bogren, H. G., et al. (1974): The variable spectrum of echocardiographic manifestations of the mitral valve prolapse syndrome. *Circulation*, 50:33–41.

100. DeMaria, A. N., Mason, D. T. (1974): "Silent" mitral prolapse—Letter to the editor. *Circulation*, 50:1285.

101. DeMaria, A. N., Neumann, A., Lee, G., et al. (1977): Echocardiographic identification of the mitral valve prolapse syndrome. *Am. J. Med.*, 62:819–829.

102. DePasquale, N. P., Burch, G. E. (1971): Papillary muscle dysfunction in coronary (ischemic) heart disease. *Ann. Rev. Med.*, 22:327–342.

103. DeSilva, R. A., Shubrooks, S. J. (1977): Mitral valve prolapse with atrioventricular and sinoatrial node abnormalities of long duration. *Am. Heart J.*, 93:772–775.

104. Desser, K. B., Benchimol, A. (1972): The apexcardiogram in patients with the syndrome of midsystolic click and late systolic murmur. *Chest*, 62:739–740.

105. Desser, K. B., Benchimol, A. (1977): External pulse recordins in combined mitral valve prolapse and obliterative cardiomyopathy. *Chest*, 71:394–395.

106. Desser, K. B., Benchimol, A. (1977): Click in the neck—unusual presentation of mitral-valve prolapse—Letter to the editor. *New Engl. J. Med.*, 297:619.

107. Desser, K. B., Promisloff, S. D., Yellen, L. G., et al. (1976): Stress electrocardiography in Uhl's anomaly with mitral valve prolapse. *Chest*, 70:529–531.

108. Devereux, R. B., Perloff, J. K., Reichek, N., et al. (1976): Mitral valve prolapse. *Circulation*, 54:3–14.

109. Dillon, J. C., Haine, C. L., Chang, S., et al. (1971): Use of echocardiography in patients with prolapsed mitral valve. *Circulation*, 43:503–507.

110. Dock, W. (1973): Production mode of systolic clicks due to mitral cusp prolapse. *Arch. Intern. Med.*, 132:118–125.

111. Duca, P. R., Gottlieb, R., Kasparian, H., et al. (1975): Abnormal myocardial lactate metabolism as an additional feature of the syndrome of mitral valve prolapse. *Am. J. Cardiol.* (*abstr*), 35:133.

112. Eber, L., Berkovits, B. V., Matloff, S. M., et al. (1974): Dynamic characterization of premature ventricular beats and ventricular tachycardias. *Am. J. Cardiol.*, 33:378–383.

113. Editorial (1975): So-called innocent systolic murmurs. *Br. Med. J.*, 5952:229–230.

114. Edwards, J. E. (1971): Clinicopathologic Correlations: Mitral insufficiency resulting from "overshooting" of leaflets. *Circulation*, 43:606–612.

115. Eguchi, S., Nakaruma, C., Asano, K., et al. (1976): Surgical treatment of floppy mitral valve syndrome in children. *J. Thor. Cardiovasc. Surg.*, 71:899–903.

116. Ehlers, K. H., Engle, M. A., Levin, A. R., et al. (1970): Left ventricular abnormality with late mitral insufficiency and abnormal electrocardiogram. *Am. J. Cardiol.*, 26:333–340.

117. Embi, A., Aranda, J., Scherlag, B. J., et al. (1975): Induction of mitral valve prolapse in the dog with one and two vessel stenosis. *Circulation* (*abstr*), 51,52 (Suppl II):178.

118. Epstein, E. J., Coulshed, N. (1973): Phonocardiogram and apex cardiogram in systolic click—late systolic murmur syndrome. *Br. Heart J.*, 35:260–275.

119. Evans, P., Hughes, D., Smith, S., et al. (1976): Joint laxity associated with the mitral valve prolapse syndrome. *Circulation* (*abstr*), 53,54 (Suppl II):103.

120. Facquet, J., Alhomme, P., Raharison, S. (1964): Sur la signification du souffle frequemment associe au claquement telesystolique. *Acta Cardiol.*, 19:417–422.

121. Farry, J. P., Simon, A. L., Ross, A. M., et al. (1975): Quantitative angiographic assessment of the mitral annulus in the prolapsing leaflet syndrome. *Circulation* (*abstr*), 51,52 (Suppl II): 12.

122. Fasola, A. F., Noble, R. J., Zipes, D. P. (1977): Treatment of recurrent ventricular tachycardia and fibrillation with aprindine. *Am. J. Cardiol.*, 39:903–910.

123. Feigenbaum, H. (1976): *Echocardiography*, 2nd edition. Lea & Febiger, Philadelphia.

124. Feldman, M. I., ElsSaid, G., Garcia, E., et al. (1972): Early non-ejection clicks:

A variant of the auscultatory electrocardiographic syndrome. *Ann. Intern. Med.,* 76:868.

125. Felner, J. M., Harwood, S., Mond, H., et al. (1977): Systolic honks in young children. *Am. J. Cardiol.,* 40:206–211.
126. Fernex, M., Fernex, C. (1958): La degenerescence mucoide des valvules mitrales. Ses repercussions fonctionnelles. *Helv. Med. Acta.,* 25:694–705.
127. Fontana, M. E., Kissell, G. L., Criley, J. M. (1975): Functional anatomy of mitral valve prolapse—Physiologic Principles of Heart Sounds and Murmurs. *American Heart Association Monograph* No. 46, pp. 126–132.
128. Fontana, M. E., Pence, H. L., Leighton, R. F., et al. (1970): The varying clinical spectrum of the systolic click-late systolic murmur syndrome. *Circulation,* 41:807–816.
129. Fontana, M. E., Wooley, C. F., Leighton, R. F., et al. (1975): Postural changes in left ventricular and mitral valvular dynamics in the systolic click-late systolic murmur syndrome. *Circulation,* 51:165–173.
130. Frable, W. J. (1969): Mucinous degeneration of the cardiac valves. *J. Thorac. Cardiovasc. Surg.,* 58:62–70.
131. French, J. W., Baum, D., Popp, R. I. (1975): Echocardiographic findings in Uhl's anomaly. *Am. J. Cardiol.,* 36:349–353.
132. Friesinger, G. C., Biern, R. O., Likar, I., et al. (1972): Exercise electrocardiography and vasoregulatory abnormalities. *Am. J. Cardiol.,* 30:733–740.
133. Gallagher, J. J., Gilbert, M., Stevenson, R. H., et al. (1975): Wolff-Parkinson White syndrome. The problem, evaluation and surgical correction. *Circulation,* 51:767.
134. Gallagher, J. J., Pritchett, E. L. C., Benditt, D. G., et al. (1977): High dose disopyramide phosphate: An effective treatment for refractory ventricular tachycardia. *Circulation (abstr),* 55,56 (Suppl III):225.
135. Gallagher, J. J., Pritchett, E. L. C., Sealy, W. C., et al. (1977): Tpe A WPW and mitral valve prolapse—Letter to the editor. *Circulation,* 56:137.
136. Gallavardin, L. (1932): Nouvelle observation avec autopsie d'un pseudodedoublement du 2e bruit de coeur simulant le dedoublement mitral. *La Prat. Med. Franc.,* 13:19.
137. Gentzler, R. D., Gault, J. H., Liedtke, A. J., et al. (1975): Congenital absence of the left circumflex coronary artery in the systolic click syndrome. *Circulation,* 52:490–496.
138. Gilbert, B. W., Schatz, R. A., VonRamm, O. T., et al. (1976): Mitral valve prolapse. Two-dimensional echocardiographic and angiographic correlation. *Circulation,* 54:716–723.
139. Girard, D. E., Girard, J. B. (1977): Mitral valve prolapse-click syndrome in twins. *Am. Heart J.,* 94:813–815.
140. Glassman, E., Kronzon, I. (1974): Coronary artery distribution in patients with prolapse of the mitral valve. *Circulation (abstr),* 49,50 (Suppl III):228.
141. Goodman, D. J., Harrison, D. C., Popp, R. L. (1974): Echocardiographic features of primary pulmonary hypertension. *Am. J. Cardiol.,* 33:438–443.
142. Goodman, D., Kimbiris, D., Linhart, J. W. (1974): Chordae tendineae rupture complicating the systolic click-late systolic murmur syndrome. *Am. J. Cardiol.,* 33:681–684.
143. Gooch, A. S., Maranhao, V., Scampardonis, G., et al. (1972): Prolapse of both mitral and tricuspid leaflets in systolic murmur-click syndrome. *New Engl. J. Med.,* 287:1218–1222.
144. Gooch, A. S., Vicencio, F., Maranhao, et al. (1972): Arrhythmias and left ventricular asynergy in the prolapsing mitral leaflet syndrome. *Am. J. Cardiol.,* 29:611–620.
145. Gramiak, R., Waag, R. C. (1975): Cardiac ultrasound. Mosby, Saint Louis.
146. Greenwald, J. G. (1974): "Silent" mitral prolapse—Letter to the editor. *Circulation,* 50:1284–1285.
147. Griffith, J. P. C. (1892): Mid-systolic and late-systolic mitral murmurs. *Am. J. Med. Sci.,* 104:285–294.
148. Grossman, H., Fleming, R. J., Engle, M. A., et al. (1968): Angiocardiography

in the apical systolic click syndrome: Left ventricular abnormality, mitral insufficiency, late systolic murmur, and inversion of T waves. *Radiology, 91*:898–904.

149. Gulotta, S. J., Gulco, L., Padmanabhan, et al. (1974): The syndrome of systolic click, murmur and mitral valve prolapse—a cardiomyopathy? *Circulation, 49*:717–728.

150. Guthrie, R. B., Edwards, J. E. (1976): Pathology of the myxomatous mitral valve. Nature, secondary changes and complications. *Minn. Med., 59*:637–647.

151. Haas, J. M. (1976): The effect of pregnancy on the midsystolic click and murmur of the prolapsing posterior leaflet of the mitral valve. *Am. Heart J., 92*:407–408.

152. Halberstam, M. (1976): *The New York Times*, September 5, 1976.

153. Halberstam, M. J. (1976): Systolic click—is it a syndrome, a diagnostic sign, or a benign curiosity? *Modern Med.,* Oct. 15:59–60.

154. Hancock, E. W., Cohn, K. (1966): The syndrome associated with midsystolic click and late systolic murmur. *Am. J. Med., 41*:183–196.

155. Heikkila, J. (1967): Mitral incompetence as a complication of acute myocardial infarction. *Acta. Med. Scand.* (Suppl) 475:

156. Higgins, C. B., Reinke, R. T., Gosink, B. B., et al. (1976): The significance of mitral valve prolapse in middle-aged and elderly men. *Am. Heart J., 91*:292–296.

157. Hill, D. G., Davies, M. J., Braimbridge, M. V. (1974): The natural history and surgical management of the redundant cusp syndrome (floppy mitral valve). *J. Thorac. Cardiovasc. Surg., 67*:519–525.

158. Horgan, J. H., Beachley, M. C., Robinson, F. D. (1975): Tricuspid valve prolapse diagnosed by echocardiogram. *Chest, 68*:822–824.

159. Howard, P. F., Desser, K. B., Benchimol, A. (1977): Systolic retraction of the aortic valve in mitral valve prolapse. *Chest, 71*:659–660.

160. Humphries, W. C., Hammer, W. J., McDonough, M. T., et al. (1977): Echocardiographic equivalents of a flail mitral leaflet. *Am. J. Cardiol., 40*:802–807.

161. Humphries, J. O., Mckusick, V. A. (1962): The differentiation of organic and "innocent" systolic murmurs. *Prog. Cardiovasc. Dis., 5*:152–171.

162. Hunt, D., Sloman, G. (1969): Prolapse of the posterior leaflet of the mitral valve occurring in eleven members of a family. *Am. Heart J., 78*:149–153.

163. Hutter, A. M., Dinsmore, R. E., Willerson, J. T., et al. (1971): Early systolic clicks due to mitral valve prolapse. *Circulation, 44*:516–522.

164. Hynes, K. M., Frye, R. L., Brandenburg, R. O., et al. (1974): Atrial septal defect (secundum) associated with mitral regurgitation. *Am. J. Cardiol., 34*:333–338.

165. Jacobs, W. F., Battle, W. E., Ronan, J. A. (1974): False-positive ST-T-wave changes secondary to hyperventilation and exercise. *Ann. Intern. Med., 81*:479–482.

166. Jacobs, W. R., Talano, J. V., Stephanides, L. (1977): Palpitations and late systolic murmur in a young man. *Arch. Intern. Med., 137*:911–913.

167. James, T. N. (1967): Pathology of small coronary arteries. *Am. J. Cardiol., 20*:679.

168. Jamshidi, A., Robbenhaar, J. K. (1970): Myxomatous transformation of the aortic and mitral valve with subaortic "Sail-Like" membrane. *Am. J. Med., 49*:114–117.

169. Jeresaty, R. M. (1971): The syndrome associated with mid-systolic click and/or late systolic murmur: Analysis of 32 cases. *Chest, 59*:643–647.

170. Jeresaty, R. M. (1971): Mitral ballooning—a possible mechanism of mitral insufficiency in diseases associated with reduced end-systolic volume of the left ventricle. *Chest, 60*:114–115.

171. Jeresaty, R. M. (1971): Ballooning of the mitral valve leaflets angiographic study of 24 patients. *Radiology, 100*:45–52.

172. Jeresaty, R. M., Liss, J. P. (1972): Midsystolic clicks and coronary artery disease—Letter to the editor. *Circulation, 45*:1145.

173. Jeresaty, R. M. (1972): Prolapse of the anterior mitral leaflet: A new angiographic sign. *Circulation (abstr),* 45,46 (Suppl II):

174. Jeresaty, R. M., Liss, J. P. (1973): Midsystolic clicks and coronary heart disease—Letter to the editor. *Chest, 63*:297–298.

175. Jeresaty, R. M. (1973): Mitral valve prolapse-click syndrome. *Progr. Cardiovasc. Dis., 15*:623–652.

176. Jeresaty, R. M. (1974): Mitral valve prolapse—Letter to the editor. *Circulation,* 49:1267–1268.
177. Jeresaty, R. M. (1974): Atrial septal defect and myxomatous mitral valve prolapse —Letter to the editor. *New Engl. J. Med.,* 290:1088.
178. Jeresaty, R. M., Landry, A. B., Liss, J. P. (1975): Silent mitral valve prolapse: analysis of 32 cases. *Am. J. Cardiol.,* 35:146.
179. Jeresaty, R. M. (1975): Etiology of the mitral valve prolapse-click syndrome. *Am. J. Cardiol.,* 36:109–113.
180. Jeresaty, R. M. (1975): Mitral Valve prolapse-click syndrome in atrial septal defect. *Chest,* 67:132–133.
181. Jeresaty, R. M. (1976): Mitral valve prolapse clicks—What they mean. *Primary Cardiol,* 2:20–23.
182. Jeresaty, R. M. (1977): Mitral valve prolapse in patients with coronary artery disease—correspondence. *Br. Heart J.,* 39:1043.
183. Josephson, M. E., Horowitz, L. N., Kastor, J. A. (1977): Paroxysmal supraventricular tachycardia in patients with mitral valve prolapse. *Circulation,* 57:111– 115.
184. Jugdutt, B., Basualdo, C., Freeman, H., et al. (1976): Acromegaly, the systolic click syndrome, and Group D streptococcal endocarditis. *Chest,* 69:690–692.
185. Kaufmann, R., Theophile, U. (1967): Automatie-fordernde denungseffekte und purkinjefaden, papillarmuskeln und vorhoftrabekeln von Rhesus-Affen, Pfluegers. *Arch.* 197:174, (includes summary in English).
186. Kawai, N., Kimbiris, D., Segal, B. (1971): Pure mitral insufficiency and prolapsed mitral valve. *Chest (abstr),* 60:295.
187. Keck, E. W., Henschel, W. G., Gruhl, L. (1976): Mitral valve prolapse in children with secundum type atrial septal defect (ASD II). *Eur. J. Pediatr.,* 121:89–97.
188. Keenan, T. J., Schwartz, M. J. (1973): Tricuspid whoop. *Am. J. Cardiol.,* 31:642– 645.
189. Kendall, M. E., Rembert, J. C., Greenfield, J. C. (1973): Pressure-flow studies in man: The nature of the aortic flow pattern in both valvular mitral insufficiency and the prolapsing mitral valve syndrome. *Am. Heart J.,* 86:359–365.
190. Kerber, R. E., Harrison, D. C. (1972): Paradoxical electrocardiographic effects on amyl nitrite in coronary artery disease. *Br. Heart J.,* 34:851–857.
191. Kerber, R. E., Lsaeff, D. M., Hancock, E. W. (1971): Echocardiographic patterns in patients with the syndrome of systolic click and late systolic murmur. *N. Engl. J. Med.,* 284:691–693.
192. Kerin, N. Z., Edelstein, J., Louridas, G. (1976): Prolapsing mitral valve leaflet syndrome. A spectrum that includes cleft posterior mitral valve. *Cathet. Cardiovasc. Diagn.,* 2:77–85.
193. Kern, W. H., Tucher, B. L. (1972): Myxoid changes in cardiac valves: pathologic, clinical, and ultrastructural studies. *Am. Heart J.,* 84:294–301.
194. Khullar, S. C., Leighton, R. F. (1974): Myocardial lactate production in mitral valve prolapse syndrome. *Circulation (abstr),* 49,50:(Suppl III):232.
195. Killebrew, E., Cohn, K. (1971): Observations on murmurs originating from incompetent heterograft mitral valves. *Am. Heart J.,* 81:490–493.
196. Kincaid, D. T., Botti, R. E. (1974): Subacute bacterial endocarditis in a patient with isolated, nonejection systolic click but without a murmur. *Chest,* 66:88–89.
197. Kittredge, R. D., Shimomura, S., Cameron, A., et al. (1970): Prolapsing mitral valve leaflets: Cineangiographic demonstration. *Am. J. Roentgen.,* 109:84–93.
198. Klein, G., Kostuk, W. J., Chamberlain, M. J. (1977): Stress myocardial scinitgraphy in patients with mitral leaflet prolapse. *Circulation,* 55,56 (Suppl III):217.
199. Koch, F. H., Billingham, M. E., Mason, J. W., et al. (1977): Pathogenesis of the click-murmur prolapse syndrome. Biopsy evidence supporting an underlying cardiomyopathic process. *Am. J. Cardiol.,* 39:272.
200. Koch, F. H., Billingham, M. E., Rider, A. K., et al. (1976): Pathophysiology of "angina" with normal coronary angiograms. *Circulation,* 54:(Suppl II):173.
201. Koch, F. H., Hancock, E. W. (1976): Ten year follow-up of forty patients with the mid-systolic click/late systolic mummur syndrome. *Am. J. Cardiol. (abstr),* 37:149.

202. Kostich, N. K., Opitz, J. M. (1965): Ullrich-Turner syndrome associated with cystic medial necrosis of the aorta and great vessels. *Am. J. Med.,* 38:943–950.
203. Kostuk, W. J., Barnett, H. J. M., Silver, M. D. (1977): Strokes: A complication of mitral-leaflet prolapse? *Lancet,* I:313–316.
204. Kraus, M. E., Naughton, J. (1976): Effect of exercise on left ventricular ejection time in patients with prolapsing mitral leaflet syndrome. *Chest,* 69:484–489.
205. Kreisman, K., Kleiger, R., Schad, N., et al. (1971): Arrhythmia in prolapse of the mitral valve. *Circulation,* 43,44 (Suppl II):44.
206. Kremkau, E. L., Gilbertson, P. R., Bristow, J. D. (1973): Acquired, nonrheumatic mitral regurgitation: Clinical management with emphasis on evaluation of myocardial performance. *Prog. Cardiovasc. Dis.,* 15:403–425.
207. Krikler, D., Curry, P., Kafetz, K. (1976): Pre-excitation and mitral valve prolapse. *Br. Med. J.,* I:1257.
208. Kuhn, C., Weber, N. (1973): Mural bacterial endocarditis of a ventricular friction lesion. *Arch. Pathol.,* 95:92–93.
209. Lababidi, Z. (1976): Floppy mitral whistle heard across the room—Letter to the editor. *Am. Heart J.,* 91:825.
210. Lachman, A. S., Bramwell-Jones, D. M., Lakier, J. B., et al. (1975): Infective endocarditis in the billowing mitral leaflet syndrome. *Br. Heart J.,* 37:326–330.
211. Lardani, H., Moreyra, A., Manubens, S., et al. (1976): Electrocardiographic findings in 125 patients with idiopathic prolapse of the mitral valve studied by angiography. *Cleveland Clin. Q.,* 43:181–194.
212. Leachman, R. D., De Francheschi, A., Zamalloa, O. (1969): Late systolic murmurs and clicks associated with abnormal mitral valve ring. *Am. J. Cardiol.,* 23:679–683.
213. Leachman, R. D., Cokkinos, E. V., Cooley, D. A. (1976): Association of ostium secundum atrial septal defects with mitral valve prolapse. *Am. J. Cardiol.,* 38:167–169.
214. Leatham, A. (1958): Auscultation of the heart. *Lancet,* 2:703–757.
215. Leatherman, L. L., Armbrust, C. A., Hall, R. J., et al. (1973): Chest pain and abnormal postexercise ECG's with normal coronary arteriograms in patients with click-late systolic murmur syndrome. *Tex. Med.,* 69:44–48.
216. Lebauer, E. J., Perloff, J. K., Keliher, T. F. (1967): The isolated systolic click with bacterial endocarditis. *Am. Heart J.,* 73:534–537.
217. Leichtman, D., Nelson, R., Gobel, F. L., et al. (1976): Bradycardia with mitral valve prolapse. *Ann. Intern. Med.,* 85:453–457.
218. Leon, D. F., Leonard, J. J., Kroetz, F. W., et al. (1966): Late systolic murmurs, clicks, and whoops arising from the mitral valve. *Am. Heart J.,* 72:325–336.
219. Lesch, M. (1976): Mitral-valve prolapse: A clinical spectrum (editorial). *New Engl. J. Med.,* 294:1117–1118.
220. LeWinter, M. M., Hoffman, J. R., Shell, W. E., et al. (1974): Phenylephrine-induced atypical chest pain in patients with prolapsing mitral valve leaflets. *Am. J. Cardiol.,* 34:12–18.
221. Lewis, H. P. (1971): Midsystolic clicks and coronary heart disease. *Circulation,* 44:493–494.
222. Liedtke, A. J., Gault, J. H., Leaman, D. M., et al. (1973): Geometry of left ventricular contraction in the systolic click syndrome. Characterization of a segmental myocardial abnormality. *Circulation,* 47:27–35.
223. Lillie, R. B. (1965): Histopathologic Technique and Practical Histochemistry, 3rd edition, pp. 493–495. McGraw-Hill, New York.
224. Litwak, R. (1977): Personal communication.
225. Linhart, J. W., Taylor, W. J. (1966): The late apical systolic murmur. *Am. J. Cardiol.,* 18:164–168.
226. Lobstein, H. P., Horowitz, L. D., Curry, G. C., et al. (1973): Electrocardiographic abnormalities and coronary arteriograms in the mitral click-murmur syndrome. *New Engl. J. Med.,* 289:127–131.
227. Longo, M. R., Froelicher, V. F., Strom, J., et al. (1977): Investigating the arrhythmic nature of prolapsing mitral leaflet syndrome. *Chest,* 72:3.

228. Lown, B., Graboys, T. B. (1977): Management of patients with malignant ventricular arrhythmias. *Am. J. Cardiol.*, 39:910–918.
229. Luxton, M., Peter, T., Hunt, D., et al. (1975): The floppy mitral valve syndrome. A review of fourteen patients requiring valve surgery. *Aust. NZ J. Med.*, 5:112–116.
230. Malcolm, A. D., Ahuja, S. P. (1975): Unusual ECG response to exercise patients with mitral prolapse. *Circulation (abstr)*, 52 (Suppl II): 114.
231. Malcolm, A. D., Bonghaner, D. R., Kostuk, W. J., et al. (1976): Clinical features and investigative findings in presence of mitral leaflet prolapse. Study of 85 consecutive patients. *Br. Heart J.*, 38:244–256.
232. Maranhao, V., Gooch, A. S., Yang, S. S., et al. (1975): Prolapse of the tricuspid leaflets in the systolic murmur-click syndrome. *Cathet. Cardiovasc. Diagn.*, I:81–90.
233. Markiewicz, W., Stoner, J., London, E., et al. (1976): Mitral valve prolapse in one hundred presumably healthy young females. *Circulation*, 53:64–473.
234. Martin, C. (1975): Mid-systolic click, late systolic murmur syndrome associated with complete heart block. *J. Electrocardiol.*, 8:191–194.
235. Martin, C. E., Hufnagel, C. A., deLeon, A. C. (1969): Calcified atria myxoma: Diagnostic significance of the "systolic tumor sound" in a case presenting as tricuspid insufficiency. *Am. Heart J.*, 78:245–250.
236. Mathey, D. G., Decoodt, P. R., Allen, H. N., et al. (1977): Abnormal left ventricular contraction pattern in the systolic click-late systolic murmur syndrome. *Circulation*, 56:311–315.
237. Marchand, P., Barlow, B., DuPlessis, L. A., et al. (1966): Mitral regurgitation with rupture of normal chordate tendineae. *Br. Heart J.*, 28:746–758.
238. Markiewicz, W., Stoner, J. London, E., et al. (1976): Effect of transducer placement on echocardiographic mitral valve systolic motion. *Eur. J. Cardiol.*, 4/3:359–366.
239. Marshall, C. E., Shappel, S. D. (1974): Sudden death and the ballooning posterior leaflet syndrome: detailed anatomic and histochemical investigation. *Arch. Pathol.*, 98:134–138.
240. Massie, B., Botvinick, E. H., Shames, D., et al. (1978): Myocardial perfusion scintigraphy in patients with mitral valve prolapse. *Circulation*, 57:19–26.
241. Mathews, E., Henry, W. L., Ronan, J. A., et al. (1976): Two dimensional echo evaluation of mitral valve prolapse—an explanation of the patterns seen with M-mode echocardiograms. *Circulation (abstr)*, 53,54 (Suppl II): 234.
242. Mathey, D. G., Decoodt, P. R., Allen, H. N., et al. (1976): The determinants of onset of mitral valve prolapse in the systolic click-late systolic murmur syndrome. *Circulation*, 53:872–878.
243. McDonald, A., Harris, A., Jefferson, K., et al. (1971): Association of prolapse of posterior cusp of mitral valve and atrial septal defect. *Br. Heart J.*, 33:383–387.
244. McKay, R., Yacoub, N. H. (1973): Clinical and pathological findings in patients with "floppy" valves treated surgically. *Circulation*, 47,48 (Suppl III):63–73.
245. McKay, R., Yacoub, M. H. (1976): Acute aortic dissection and medial degeneration in patients with "floppy" mitral valves. *Thorax*, 31:49–54.
246. McKusick, V. A. (1958): *Cardiovascular Sound in Health and Disease*. Williams & Wilkins, Baltimore. p. 202.
247. McKusick, V. A. (1974): Multiple forms of the Ehlers-Danlos syndrome. *Arch. Surg.*, 109:475–476.
248. McLaughlin, P., Huckell, V., Stanioff, H., et al. (1977): Exercise induced chest pain, myocardial perfusion and stress electrocardiography in patients with mitral valve prolapse. *Circulation (abstr)*, 55,56 (Suppl III):216.
249. McLaren, M. J., Hawkins, D. M., Lachman, A. S., et al. (1976): Non-ejection systolic clicks and mitral systolic murmurs in black schoolchildren of Soweto, Johannesburg. *Br. Heart J.*, XXXVIII:718–724.
250. Mercer, E. N., Frye, R. L., Giuliani, E. R. (1970): Late systolic click in non-obstructive cardiomyopathy. *Br. Heart J.*, 32:691–695.
251. Meyer, J. F., Frank, M. J., Goldberg, S., et al. (1977): Systolic mitral flutter, an echocardiographic clue to the diagnosis of ruptured chordae tendineae. *Am. Heart J.*, 93:3–8.

252. Miller, A. B., Salcedo, E. E., Bahler, R. C. (1975): Prolapsed mitral valve associated with the Holt-Oram syndrome. *Chest,* 67:230–232.
253. Mills, P., Rose, J., Hollingsworth, B. A., et al. (1977): Long-term prognosis of mitral-valve prolapse. *New Engl. J. Med.,* 297:13–18.
254. Millward, D. K., McLaurin, L. P., Craige, E. (1973): Echocardiographic studies to explain opening snaps in presence of nonstenotic mitral valves. *Am. J. Cardiol.,* 31:64–70.
255. Morcerf, F., Salcedo, E. E., Siegel, W. (1976): Echocardiographic determination of the etiology of severe mitral regurgitation. *Clev Clin. Q.,* 43:163–174.
256. Myburgh, D. H. (1969): The effect of amyl nitrite on the electrocardiogram of normal subjects. *S. Afr. Med. J.,* 43:517.
257. Myers, M. G., Buda, A. J., Levene, D. L., et al. (1976): Coronary-artery spasm and mitral-valve prolapse. *Lancet,* I:864.
258. Naggar, C. Z., Alexander, S. (1976): Propranolol treatment of VPB'S—Letter to the editor. *New Engl. J. Med.,* 294:903–904.
259. Nakhjavan, F. K., Natarajan, G., Seshachary, P., et al. (1976): The relationship between prolapsing mitral leaflet syndrome and angina and normal coronary arteriograms. *Chest,* 70:706–710.
260. Nasrallah, A. T., El-Said, G. M., Garcia, E., et al. (1974): Early nonejection systolic clicks. *Tex. Med.,* 70:82–85.
261. Natarajan, G., Nakhjavan, F. K., Kahn, D., et al. (1975): Myocardial metabolic studies in prolapsing mitral leaflet syndrome. *Circulation,* 52:1105–1110.
262. Nichol, P. M., Gilbert, B. W., Kisslo, J. A. (1977): Two-dimensional echocardiographic assessment of mitral stenosis. *Circulation,* 55:120–128.
263. Nutter, D. O., Wickliffe, C., Gilbert, C. A., et al. (1975): The pathophysiology of idopathic mitral valve prolapse. *Circulation,* 52:295–305.
264. O'Rourke, R. A., Crawford, M. H. (1976): The systolic click-murmur syndrome: Clinical recognition and management. *Curr. Prob. Cardiol.,* I:1–60.
265. Osler, W. (1879–1880): On a remarkable heart murmur heard at a distance from the chest wall. *Can. Med. Surg. J.,* 8:518–519.
266. Owens, J. S., Kotler, M. N., Segal, B. L., et al. (1976): Pseudoprolapse of the mitral valve in a patient with pericardial effusion. *Chest,* 69:214–215.
267. Owens, J. P., Williams, R. G., Fellows, K. E. (1974): Prolapsing mitral leaflet associated with secundum atrial septal defect. *Circulation (abstr),* 50 (Suppl III): 240.
268. Padmanabhan, V., Margouleff, D., Binder, A., et al. (1977): Thallium-201 myocardial imaging during exercise in mitral valve prolapse. *Circulation (abstr),* 55,56 (Suppl III):217.
269. Pandian, M. G., Lichtman, A. (1976): Mitral valve prolapze and bacterial endocarditis. *Conn. Med.,* 40:675–676.
270. Pasternak, A., Gervais, A. R., Gueret, P., et al. (1974): The systolic click syndrome: Myocardial metabolism, contraction abnormalities and ventricular performance. *Circulation (abstr),* 50:Suppl III:239.
271. Payvandi, M. N., Kerber, R. E., Phelps, G. D., et al. (1977): Cardiac, skeletal and ophthalmologic abnormalities in relatives of patients with the Marfan syndrome. *Circulation,* 55:797–802.
272. Perloff, J. K. (1977): Mitral valve prolapse and noncardiac symptoms—Letter to the editor. *Circulation,* 55:680.
273. Pickering, D., Keith, J. D. (1971): Systolic clicks with ventricular septal defects. A sign of aneurysm of ventricular septum? *Br. Heart J.,* 33:538–539.
274. Pieroni, D. R., Bell, B. B., Krovetz, L. J., et al. (1971): Auscultatroy recognition of aneurysm of the membranous ventricular septum associated with small ventricular septal defect. *Circulation,* 44:733–739.
275. Pocock, W. A., Barlow, J. B. (1970): Postexercise arrhtthmias in the billowing posterior mitral leaflet syndrome. *Am. Heart J.,* 80:740–745.
276. Pocock, W. A., Barlow, J. B. (1971): Etiology and electrocardiographic features of the billowing posterior mitral leaflet syndrome: Analysis of a further 130 patients with a late systolic murmur or nonejection systolic click. *Am. J. Med.,* 51:731–739.

277. Pocock, W. A., Lakier, J. B., Hitchcock, J. F., Barlow, J. B. (1977): Mitral valve aneurysm after infective endocarditis in the billowing mitral leaflet syndrome. *Am. J. Cardiol.,* 40:130–132.

278. Pomerance, A. (1969): Ballooning deformity (Mucoid degeneration) of atrioventricular valves. *Br. Heart J.,* 31:343–351.

279. Pomerance, A. (1972): "Pathology and valvular heart disease" *Br. Heart J.,* 34: 437–443.

280. Popp, R. L. (1976): Echocardiographic assessment of cardiac disease. *Circulation,* 54:538–552.

281. Popp, R. L. (1976): Special features and new data in mitral valve echocardiography. The mitral valve: A pluridisciplinary approach. Publishing Sciences Group.

282. Popp, R. L., Brown, O. R., Silverman, J. F., et al. (1974): Echocardiographic abnormalities in the mitral valve prolapse syndrome. *Circulation,* 49:428–433.

283. Popp, R. L., Winkle, R. A. (1976): Mitral-valve prolapse syndrome. *JAMA,* 236:867–870.

284. Pridie, R. B. (1976): Echocardiography in mitral valve prolapse—Letter to the editor. *Br. Med. J.,* I:1591.

285. Procacci, P. M. (1976): Letter to the editor. Mitral-valve prolapse *New Engl. J. Med.,* 295:447.

286. Procacci, P. M., Savran, S. V., Schreiter, S. L., et al. (1976): Prevalence of clinical mitral-valve prolapse in 1169 young women. *New Engl. J. Med.,* 294: 1086–1088.

287. Rackley, C. E., Whalen, R. E., Floyd, W. L., et al. (1966): The precordial honk. *Am. J. Cardiol.,* 17:509–515.

288. Raizada, V., Benchimol, A., Desser, K. B., et al. (1977): Mitral valve prolapse in patients with coronary artery disease. Echocardiographic-angiographic correlation. *Br. Heart J.,* 39:53–60.

289. Rakowski, H., Martin, R. P., Popp, R. L. (1977): Two-dimensional echocardiographic findings in mitral valve prolapse. *Circulation (abstr),* 55,56 (Suppl III): 154.

290. Rakowski, H., Waxman, M. B., Wald, R. W., et al. (1975): Mitral valve prolapse and ventricular fibrillation. *Circulation (abstr),* 52:(Suppl II):93.

291. Ranganathan, N., Lam, J. H. C., Wigle, E. D., et al. (1970): Morphology of the human mitral valve. II. The valve leaflets. *Circulation,* 41:459.

292. Ranganathan, N., Silver, M. D., Robinson, T. I., et al. (1973): Angiographic-morphologic correlation in patients with severe mitral regurgitation due to prolapse of the posterior mitral valve leaflet. *Circulation,* 48:514–518.

293. Ranganathan, N., Silver, M. D., Robinson, T. I., et al. (1976): Idiopathic prolapsed mitral leaflet syndrome. *Circulation,* 54:707–716.

294. Ranganathan, N., Silver, M. D., Wigle, E. D. (1974): Mitral valve prolapse. *Circulation,* 49:1268–1269.

295. Ranganathan, N., Silver, M. D., Wigle, E. D. (1976): Recent advances in the knowledge of the anatomy of the mitral valve. The mitral valve: A pluridisciplinary approach. Publishing Sciences Group.

296. Read, R. C., Thal, A. P. (1966): Surgical experience with symptomatic myxomatous valvular transformation (the floppy valve syndrome). *Surgery,* 59:173–182.

297. Read, R. C., Thal, A. P., Wendy, V. E. (1965): Symptomatic valvular myxomatous transformation (the floppy valve syndrome): A possible Forme Fruste of the Marfan Syndrome. *Circulation,* 32:897–910.

298. Reid, J. V. O. (1961): Midsystolic clicks. *South African Med.,* 135:353–355.

299. Reeves, W., Griggs, R., Nanda, N. C., et al. (1976): Echocardiographic demonstration of mitral valve prolapse in muscular dystrophy. *Circulation (abstr),* 54 Suppl II):97.

300. Reiffel, J. A., Green, W. M., King, D. L., et al. (1977): Augmentation of auscultatory and echocardiographic mitral valve prolapse by atrial premature depolarizations. *Am. Heart J.,* 93:533–535.

301. Ritchie, J. L., Hammermeister, K. E., Kennedy, J. W. (1976): Refractory ventricu-

lar tachycardia and fibrillation in a patient with the prolapsing mitral leaflet syndrome: Successful control with overdrive pacing. *Am. J. Cardiol.,* 37:314–316.

302. Rizzon, P., Biasco, G., Brindicci, G., et al. (1973): Familial syndrome of midsystolic click and late systolic murmur. *Br. Heart J.,* XXXV:245–259.

303. Rizzon, P., Biasco, G., Campagna, G. M. (1971): The praecordial honk. *Br. Heart J.,* 33:707–715.

304. Roberts, W. C. (1976): The malfunctioning mitral valve: Morphologic features. *Proc. New Engl. Cardiovasc. Soc.,* 27:7–8.

305. Roberts, W. C. (1977): Personal communication.

306. Roberts, W. C., Dangel, J. C., Bulkley, B. H. (1973): Nonrheumatic valvular cardiac disease: A clinicopathologic survey of 27 different conditions causing valvular dysfunction. *Cardiovasc. Clin.,* 5:334–446.

307. Roberts, W. C., Glancy, D. L., Seningen, R. P., et al. (1976): Prolapse of the mitral valve (floppy valve) associated with Ebstein's anomaly of the tricuspid valve. *Am. J. Cardiol.,* 38:377–382.

308. Roberts, W. C., Perfoff, J. K. (1972): Mitral valvular disease—A clinicopathologic survey of the conditions causing the mitral valve to function abnormally. *Ann. Intern. Med.,* 77:939–975.

309. Roelandt, J., Willems, J., van der Hauwaert, L. G., et al. (1969): Clicks and sounds (whoops) in left sided pneumothorax. *Dis. Chest,* 56:31–36.

310. Ronan, J. A. (1975): Effect of vasoactive drugs and maneuvers on heart murmurs. Physiologic principles of heart sounds and murmurs. American Heart Association Monograph No. 46.

311. Ronan, J. A., Perloff, J. K., Harvey, W. P. (1965): Systolic clicks and the late systolic murmur, Intracardiac phonocardiographic evidence of their mitral valve origin. *Am. Heart J.,* 70:319–325.

312. Ross, R. S., Criley, J. M. (1962): Contrast radiography in mitral regurgitation. *Prog. Cardiovasc. Dis.,* 5:195–215.

313. Roy, P., Tajik, A. J., Giuliani, E. R., et al. (1976): Spectrum of echocardiographic findings in bacterial endocarditis. *Circulation,* 53:474–482.

314. Ruwitch, J. F., Weiss, A. N., Fleg, J. L., et al. (1977): Insensitivity of echocardiography in detecting mitral valve prolapse in older patients with chest pain. *Am. J. Cardiol.,* 40:686–690.

315. Sahn, D. J., Allen, H. D., Goldberg, S. J., et al. (1976): Mitral valve prolapse in children. A problem defined by real-time cross-sectional echocardiography. *Circulation,* 53:651–657.

316. Sahn, D. J., Wood, J., Allen, H. D., et al. (1977): Echocardiographic spectrum of mitral valve motion in children with and without mitral valve prolapse: The nature of false positive diagnosis. *Am. J. Cardiol.,* 39:422–431.

317. Salazar, A. E., Edwards, J. E. (1970): Friction lesions of ventricular endocardium: relation to chordae tendineae of mitral valve. *Arch. Pat.,* 90:364–376.

318. Salomon, J., Shah, P. M., Heinle, R. A. (1975): Thoracic skeletal abnormalities in idiopathic mitral valve prolapse. *Am. J. Cardiol.,* 36:32–36.

319. Salomon, N. W., Stinson, E. B., Griepp, R. B., et al. (1976): Surgical treatment of degenerative mitral regurgitation. *Am. J. Cardiol.,* 38:463–468.

320. Sasse, L. (1977): Systolic clicks and murmurs—Letter to the editor. *Am. Heart J.,* 94:265.

321. Schaal, S. F., Fontana, M. E., Wooley, C. F. (1974): Mitral valve prolapse syndrome-spectrum of conduction defects and arrhythmias. *Circulation (abstr),* 50 (Suppl III):97.

322. Scampardonis, G., Yang, S. S., Maranhao, V., et al. (1973): Left ventricular abnormalities in prolapsed mitral leaflet syndrome: review of 87 cases. *Circulation,* 48:287–297.

323. Schatz, J. W., Fischer, J. A. (1974): Paradoxic coronary embolism in a patient with mid-systolic click syndrome. *Chest,* 66:587–590.

324. Scheele, W., Allen, H. N., Kraus, R., et al. (1977): Familial prevalence and genetic transmission of mitral valve prolapse (MVP). *Circulation,* 55,56 (Suppl III):111.

325. Schwarz, D. C., Daoud, G., Kaplan, S. (1968): Dysfunction of the mitral apparatus in children. *Am. J. Cardiol.*, 21:114.
326. Schwartz, D. C., James, F. W., Kaplan, S. (1975): Exercise induced st segment depression in children with mitral valve prolapse. *Circulation (abstr)*, 52 (Suppl. II):67.
327. Schwartz, D. C., Kaplan, S., Meyer, R. A. (1975): Mitral valve prolapse in children: Clinical, echocardiographic and cine-angiographic findings in 81 cases. *Am. J. Cardiol. (abstr)*, 35:169.
328. Scully, R. E., NcNeely, B. U. (1974): Case records of the Massachusetts General Hospital. *N. Engl. J. Med.*, 291:242–249.
329. Segall, H. N. (1976): Autoauscultation in a patient with floppy mitral valve syndrome—Letter to the editor. *Am. Heart J.*, 91:269–272.
330. Selzer, A., Kelly, J. J., Vannitamby, M., et al. (1967): The syndrome of mitral insufficiency due to isolated rupture of the chordae tendineae. *Am. J. Med.*, 43: 822–836.
331. Shah, P. M., Gramiak, R. (1970): Echocardiographic recognition of mitral valve prolapse. *Circulation*, 42 (Suppl III):45.
332. Shappell, S. D., Marshall, C. E., Brown, R. E., et al. (1973): Sudden death and the familial occurrence of mid-systolic click, late systolic murmur syndrome. *Circulation*, XLVIII:1128–1134.
333. Shappell, S. D., Orr, W., Gunn, C. G. (1974): The ballooning posterior leaflet syndrome: Minnesota multiphasic personality inventory profiles in symptomatic and asymptomatic groups. *Chest*, 66:690–692.
334. Shell, W. E., Walton, J. A., Clifford, M. E., et al. (1969): The familial occurrence of the syndrome of mid-late systolic click and late systolic murmur. *Circulation*, 39:327–337.
335. Sherman, E. B., Char, F., Dungan, W. T., et al. (1970): Myxomatous transformation of the mitral valve producing mitral insufficiency: Floppy valve syndrome. *Am. J. Dis. Child.*, 119:171–175.
336. Shrivastava, S., Guthrie, R. B., Edwards, J. E. (1977): Prolapse of the mitral valve. *Mod. Concepts Cardiovasc. Dis.*, XLVI 57–62.
337. Silbert, J. E. (1973): Personal communication.
338. Singh, R., Schrank, J. P., Nolan, S. P., et al. (1972): Spontaneous rupture of mitral chordae tendineae. *JAMA*, 219:189–193.
339. Sloman, J. G., Stannard, M., Hare, W. S. C., et al. (1969): Prolapse of the posterior leaflet of the mitral valve. *Isr. J. Med. Sci.*, 5:727–731.
340. Smith, E. R., Fraser, D. B., Purdy, J. W., Anderson, R. N. (1977): Angiographic diagnosis of mitral valve prolapse: Correlation with Echocardiography. *Am. J. Cardiol.*, 40:165–170.
341. Sorensen, H. D., Smith, R. F. (1975): Lethal cardiac arrhythmias in the prolapsing valve syndrome. *J. Tenn. Med. Assoc. (abstr)*, 68:667–668.
342. Spangler, R. D., Okin, J. T., Blount, G. (1973): Echocardiography in connective tissue disorders. *Am. J. Cardiol. (abstr)*, 31:
343. Spencer, W. H., Behar, V. S., Orgain, E. S. (1973): Apex cardiogram in patients with prolapsing mitral valve. *Am. J. Cardiol.*, 32:276–282.
344. Spindola-Franco, H., Bjork, L., Miller, S., et al. (1974): Prolapse of the mitral valve: Analysis of variations of the normal mitral apparatus and a description of two new angiocardiographic signs. *Circulation (abstr)*, 49,50 (Suppl III):207.
345. Sreenivasan, V. V., Liebman, J., Linton, D. S., et al. (1968): Posterior mitral regurgitation in girls possibly due to posterior papillary muscle dysfunction. *Pediatrics*, 42:276–290.
346. Stannard, M., Goble, A. J. (1967): Endocarditis and the mitral valve. *Br. Med. J.*, 4:683.
347. Stannard, M., Rigo, S. (1968): Prolapse of the posterior leaflet of the mitral valve. Chromosome studies in three sisters. *Am. Heart J.*, 75:282–283.
348. Stannard, M., Sloman, J. G. (1967): Prolapse of the posterior leaflet of the mitral valve: A clinical, familial, and cineangiographic study. *Br. Med. J.*, 3:71–74.
349. Stapleton, J. F., Harvey, W. P. (1976): Systolic sounds. *Am. Heart J.*, 91:383–393.

350. Steelman, R. B., White, R. S., Hill, J. C., et al. (1971): Midsystolic clicks in arteriosclerotic heart disease: A new facet in the clinical syndrome of papillary muscle dysfunction. *Circulation,* 44:503–515.
351. Stein, D., Kloster, F. E. (1977): Valvular heart disease in osteogensis imperfecta. *Am. Heart J.,* 94:637–641.
352. Steinfeld, L., Dimich, I., Rappaport, H., et al. (1975): Late systolic murmur of rheumatic mitral insufficiency. *Am. J. Cardiol.,* 35:397–401.
353. Steremberg, Z. (1974): Atrial septal defect and prolapse of the mitral valve. *Med. Bull. St. Vincent's Hosp., Bridgeport, Conn.* 16:18–24.
354. Swartz, M. H., Herman, M. V., Teichholz, L. E. (1976): Dermatoglyphic patterns in patients with mitral valve prolapse: A clue to pathogenesis. *Am. J. Cardiol.,* 38:588–593.
355. Swartz, M. H., Teichholz, L. E., Donoso, E. (1977): Mitral valve prolapse. A review of associated arrhythmias. *Am. J. Med.,* 62:377–389.
356. Sze, K. C., Shah, P. M. (1976): Pseudoejection sound in hypertrophic subaortic stenosis. *Circulation,* 54:504–509.
357. Tavel, M. E., Campbell, R. W., Zimmer, J. F. (1965): Late systolic murmurs and mitral regurgitation. *Am. J. Cardiol.,* 15:719–725.
358. Teichholz, L. E., Taegtmeyer, H. (1975): Mitral valve prolapse in preexcitation syndrome. *Circulation (abstr),* 52 (Suppl II):79.
359. Thomason, H. C., Miller, A. B., Hanson, K. (1976): Congenital complete atrioventricular block and prolapsing mitral valve. *Chest,* 70:539–542.
360. Thompson, W. P., Levine, S. A. (1935): Systolic gallop rhythm: A clinical study. *New Engl. J. Med.,* 213:1021–1025.
361. Towne, W. D., Fabian, J. S., Rosen, K. M., et al. (1975): Systolic prolapse of the mitral valve in Noonan's syndrome. *Am. Heart J.,* 90:499–502.
362. Towne, W. D., Rahimtoola, S. H., Rosen, K. M., et al. (1973): The apexcardiogram in patients with systolic prolapse of the mitral valve. *Chest,* 63:569–572.
363. Towne, W. D., Rahimtolla, S. H., Sinno, M. Z., et al. (1975): The effects of right atrial and ventricular pacing on the auscultatory findings in patients with mitral valve prolapse. *Circulation,* 51:988–996.
364. Trent, J. K., Adelman, A. G., Wigle, E. D., et al. (1970): Morphology of a prolapsed posterior mitral valve leaflet. *Am. Heart J.,* 79:539–543.
365. Tucker, R. B. K., Zion, M. M., Pocock, W. A., et al. (1975): Auscultatory features of hypertrophic obstructive cardiomyopathy. *S. Afr. Med. J.,* 49:179–186.
366. Tuqan, S. K., Mau, R. D., Schwartz, M. J. (1975): Anterior myocardial infarction patterns in the mitral valve prolapse-systolic click syndrome. *Am. J. Med.,* 58:719–723.
367. Upshaw, C. B. (1975): Precordial honk due to tricuspid regurgitation. *Am. J. Cardiol.,* 35:85–88.
368. Vaisrub, S. (1975): Late systolic click syndrome—Editorial. *JAMA,* 234:632.
369. Verani, M. S., Carroll, R. J., Falsetti, H. L. (1976): Mitral valve prolapse in coronary artery disease. *Am. J. Cardiol.,* 37:1–6.
370. Victorica, B. E., Elliott, L. P., Gessner, I. H. (1974): Ostium secundum atrial septal defect associated with balloon mitral valve in children. *Am. J. Cardiol.,* 33:667–673.
371. Victorica, B. E., Elliott, L. P., Gessner, I. H. (1974): Ostium secundum atrial septal defect associated with balloon mitral valve in children. *Am. J. Cardiol.,* 33:668–673.
372. Vignola, P. A., Pohost, G. M., Curfman, G. D., et al. (1976): Correlation of echocardiographic and clinical findings in patients with pericardial effusion. *Am. J. Cardiol.,* 37:701–707.
373. Wann, L. S., Dillon, J. C., Weyman, A. E., et al. (1976): Echocardiography in bacterial endocarditis. *New Engl. J. Med.,* 295:135.
374. Waters, D. D., Clark, D. W., Symbas, P. N., et al. (1977): Aortic and mitral valve replacement in a patient with osteogenesis imperfecta. *Chest,* 72:363–364.
375. Weinrauch, L. A., McDonald, D. G., DeSilva, R. A., et al. (1977): Mitral valve prolapse in rheumatic mitral stenosis. *Chest,* 72:752–756.

376. Weiss, A. N., Mimbs, J. W., Ludbrook, P. A., et al. (1975): Echocardiographic detection of mitral valve prolapse. Exclusion of false positive diagnosis and determination of inheritance. *Circulation,* 52:1091–1096.
377. Wellens, H. J. J., Duren, D. R., Lie, K. I. (1976): Observations on mechanisms of ventricular tachycardia in man. *Circulation,* 54:237–244.
378. Werner, J. A., Schiller, N. B., Frasquier, R. (1976): Clinical cardiology: Echocardiography II Thursday morning. *Circulation (abstr),* 53,54 (Suppl II):232.
379. White, P. D.: Heart disease, 1st edition, Chap. 13, MacMillan, New York.
380. Wigle, E. G., Radowski, H., Ranganathan, N., et al. (1976): Mitral valve prolapse *Ann. Rev. Med.,* 27:165–180.
381. Winkle, R. A., Goodman, D. J., Popp, R. I. (1976): Echocardiographic evaluation of propranolol therapy for mitral valve prolapse. *Br. Heart J.,* 38:129–134.
382. Willems, J., Roelandt, J., DeGeest, H., et al. (1969): Late systolic murmurs and systolic non-ejection clicks. *Acta. Cardiol. (Brux),* 24:456–481.
383. Winkle, R. A., Goodman, D. J., Popp, R. L. (1975): Simultaneous echocardiographic phonocardiographic recordings at rest and during amyl nitrite administration in patients with mitral valve prolapse. *Circulation,* 51:522–529.
384. Winkle, R. A., Lopes, M. G., Fitzgerald, J. W., et al. (1975): Arrhythmias in patients with mitral valve prolapse. *Circulation,* 52:73–81.
385. Winkle, R. A., Lopes, M. G., Goodman, D. J., et al. (1977): Propranolol for patients with mitral valve prolapse. *Am. Heart J.,* 93:422–427.
386. Winkle, R. A., Lopes, M. G., Popp, R. L., et al. (1976): Life-threatening arrhythmias in the mitral valve prolapse syndrome. *Am. J. Med.,* 60:961–967.
387. Winters, S. J., Schreiner, B., Griggs, R. C., et al. (1976): Familial mitral valve prolapse and myotonic dystrophy. *Ann. Intern. Med.,* 85:19–22.
388. Wit, A. L., Cranefield, P. F. (1976): Triggered activity in cardiac muscle fibers of the simian mitral valve. *Circulation Res.,* 38:85–98.
389. Wit, A. L., Fenoglio, J. J., Wagner, B. M., et al. (1973): Electrophysiological properties of cardiac muscle in the anterior mitral valve leaflet and the adjacent atrium in the dog. *Circ. Res.,* 32:731–745.
390. Wolf, E., Braun, K., Stern, S. (1974): Effects of beta-receptor blocking agents propranolol and practolol on ST-T changes in neurocirculatory asthenia. *Br. Heart J.,* 36:872–879.
391. Woods, S. J., Thomas, J., Braimbridge, M. V. (1973): Mitral valve disease and open heart surgery in osteogenesis imperfecta tarda. *Br. Heart J.,* 35:103–106.
392. Woodley, D., Chambers, W., Starke, H., et al. (1977): Intermittent complete atrioventricular block masquerading as epilepsy in the mitral valve prolapse syndrome. *Chest,* 72:369–372.
393. Wooley, C. F. (1975): The spectrum of tricuspid regurgitation. Physiologic Principles of Heart Sounds and murmurs. *Am. Heart Assoc. Monograph No. 46.*
394. Wooley, C. F. (1976): Where are the diseases of yesteryear? *Circulation,* 53:749–751.
395. Wukasch, D. C., Duncan, J. M., Cooley, D. A., et al. (1977): Mitral and tricuspid annuloplasty with new flexible collar prosthesis (93 cases) *Circulation,* 55,56 (Suppl III):130.
396. Yahini, J. H., Deutsch, V., Miller, H. I., et al. (1975): Nonrheumatic mitral incompetence. *Isr. J. Med. Sci.,* 11:928–967.
397. Young, D. (1977): Noisy floppy mitral valve—Letter to the editor. *Am. Heart J.,* 93:130.
398. Zeilenga, D. W., Criley, J. M. (1972): Long term arrhythmia monitoring in the prolapsed posterior leaflet syndrome (PPLS). *Circulation,* 46:Suppl II):239.
399. Zeilenga, D. W., Criley, J. M. (1973): Mitral valve dysfunction—a possible cause of arrhythmias in the prolapsed posterior leaflet syndrome. *Clin. Res. (abstr),* 21:243.
400. ZuWallack, R., Sinatra, S., Lahiri, B., Godar, T. J., Jeresaty, R. M., Liss, J. P. (1978): Pulmonary function studies in patients with mitral valve prolapse. *Submitted for publication.*
401. Prevention of bacterial endocarditis. *Circulation,* 56:139A, 1978.

Subject Index